THE
LOW
FODMAP
RECIPE BOOK

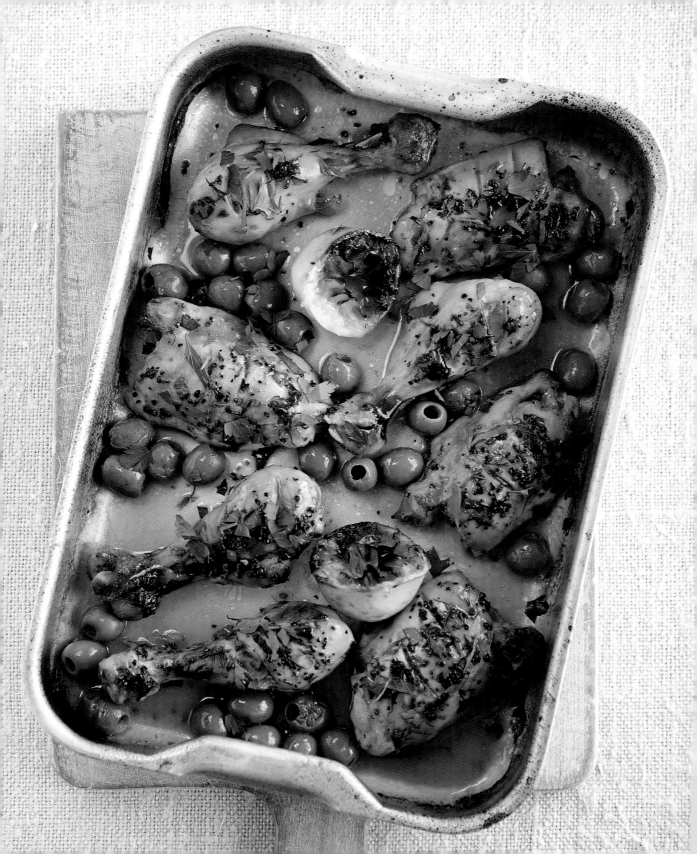

LUCY WHIGHAM

THE LOW FODMAP RECIPE BOOK

RELIEVE SYMPTOMS OF IBS, CROHN'S DISEASE & OTHER GUT DISORDERS IN 4 TO 6 WEEKS

aster

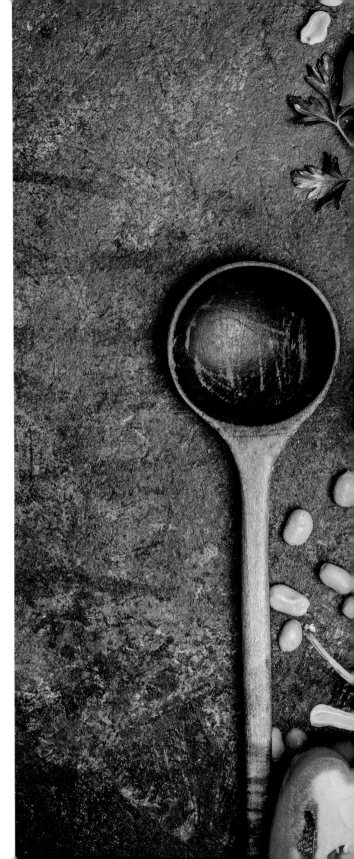

An Hachette UK Company
www.hachette.co.uk

First published in Great Britain in 2017 by Aster,
a division of Octopus Publishing Group Ltd
Carmelite House
50 Victoria Embankment
London EC4Y 0DZ
www.octopusbooks.co.uk
www.octopusbooksusa.com

Distributed in the US by Hachette Book Group
1290 Avenue of the Americas, 4th and 5th Floors
New York, NY 10020

Distributed in Canada by Canadian Manda Group
664 Annette St., Toronto, Ontario, Canada M6S 2C8

ISBN 978-1-91202-310-3

Printed and bound in China

10 9 8 7 6 5

Commissioning Editor: Leanne Bryan
Editor: Pollyanna Poulter
Senior Designer: Jaz Bahra
Designer: Geoff Fennell
Senior Production Controller: Allison Gonsalves

Disclaimer

All reasonable care has been taken in the preparation of this book
but the information it contains is not intended to take the place
treatment by a qualified medical practitioner. Before making any
changes in your health regime, always consult a physician. You must
seek professional advice if you are in any doubt about any medical
condition. Any application of the ideas and information contained
in this book is at the reader's sole discretion and risk.

Cooking notes

Standard level spoon measurements are used in all recipes.

Ovens should be preheated to the specific temperature. If using
a convection (fan-assisted) oven, follow manufacturer's instructions
for adjusting the time and the temperature.

Eggs should be medium unless otherwise stated.

This book includes dishes made with nuts and nut derivatives.

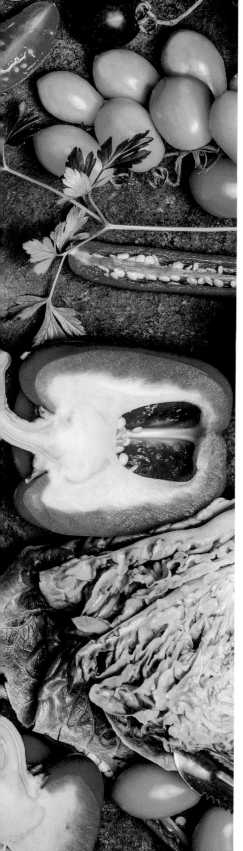

CONTENTS

INTRODUCTION

INTRODUCING THE LOW~FODMAP DIET

FODMAP is the current buzz word in the world of gut health and gastrointestinal distress. The low-FODMAP way can relieve even the most severe digestive discomfort. However, unlike most diets, this is not a fad. Rigorous clinical trials have proved the diet's effectiveness in treating symptoms of gut distress. Both the scientific community and the many people who have benefited from the diet are excited about its role in treating symptoms of IBS and other functional bowel disorders.

Around one in five people are affected by symptoms of Irritable Bowel Syndrome (IBS). Some experience the relatively mild yet disruptive symptoms of bloating and discomfort but, for others, symptoms are much more distressing, painful, and embarrassing. A number of studies have shown that IBS significantly affects the quality of life of sufferers, impacting on their enjoyment of social events, travel, and eating in restaurants, and increasing the number of days taken off work and visits to the doctor.

Medical treatments may help to ease the symptoms of IBS to some degree, but dietary manipulation is the cornerstone of treatment for the majority of people with the condition. Traditional first-line treatment involving healthy eating patterns and regular meals with adequate fluid and fiber manipulation have limited success in resolving symptoms.

The low-FODMAP diet was developed by researchers at the Monash University in Melbourne, Australia. Researchers at King's College London, in the UK, pioneered further research on its use. Clinical trials have shown that, within four to six weeks, the low-FODMAP diet results in a significant improvement of symptoms in around 75 percent of people who are diagnosed with IBS. These fantastic responses have led to the low-FODMAP diet becoming one of the mainstays of treatment for IBS worldwide, and it is considered the most effective way of treating the symptoms of IBS and other functional gut symptoms.

WHAT DOES 'FODMAP' MEAN?

FODMAP is an acronym for "fermentable oligosaccharides, disaccharides, monosaccharides, and polyols." These carbohydrates, present in a normal, healthy diet, are not fully digested and not absorbed in the small intestine and therefore go on to be fermented in the latter part of the bowel. This results in the production of gases and an influx of water, which, in susceptible individuals, causes pain, discomfort, constipation and/or diarrhea, and flatulence (gas). Lowering the intake of FODMAPs in the diet reduces the amount of gas produced and volume of water in the bowel, and can lead to substantial (many would say, miraculous) improvements in symptoms.

At first glance, the low-FODMAP diet may appear daunting because the initial stage involves entirely cutting out or greatly limiting all five families of fermentable carbohydrates to begin with. These are:

FERMENTABLE OLIGOSACCHARIDES including fructans, found in wheat, rye, onions, garlic, and various other grains and vegetables, and galacto-oligosaccharides, such as legumes

DISACCHARIDES which is lactose, found in animal milks, yogurts, and some cheeses.

MONOSACCHARIDES which refers to fructose, found in various fruits, honey, and agave nectar.

AND POLYOLS which are mannitol, sorbitol, and xylitol and are found in certain fruits.

If you have IBS or another functional bowel disorder, are looking for a way to improve your symptoms and would like to try the low-FODMAP diet, it is important to consult your doctor before embarking on the diet and to work with a registered dietitian, who will guide you through the three stages of the diet (*see* page 14).

HOW THIS BOOK CAN HELP YOU

This book provides many delicious FODMAP-friendly recipes that enable you to follow the regime while ensuring you receive a balanced, nutrient-rich diet. The recipes can be used during all stages of the diet.

There is no need to see the low-FODMAP diet as a mountain of boring restrictions. It can be something you can follow easily and with pleasure—and share with your family and friends—while your digestive symptoms diminish or even completely resolve.

Whether you need meals that are quick and easy to prepare, or you enjoy the art of cooking a dish worthy of a dinner party, this book will guide you step by step through the process of preparing tasty low-FODMAP meals. This means that you can have your cake and eat it—literally!

WHAT ARE FUNCTIONAL BOWEL DISORDERS?

THE HEALTHY GUT

The gut or gastrointestinal tract is an amazing organ that carries out an array of important functions in the body, from digestion and absorption of food to defending the body from harmful bacteria and viruses. It runs from the mouth to the anus and each section has a different job to do. After you chew and swallow your food it travels to the gut where it is broken down into individual molecules by muscular contractions in the stomach and through the release of digestive enzymes from the mouth, stomach, and small bowel. These molecules are absorbed across the gut wall into the blood stream and carried off to the liver for further processing and use in the body. Leftover waste continues down into the colon, where excess fluid and salts are reabsorbed. The rest passes out as stool.

Food is pushed through the gut by muscular contractions controlled by a complex wiring of nerve messages called the enteric nervous system. This system communicates closely with the central nervous system (the brain and spinal cord). Often referred to as the brain-gut axis, a delicate balance exists between the two systems.

Tens of trillions of bacteria, of more than a thousand species, live in the gut. One-third of these species is common to most people, while two-thirds are specific to each individual (much like our individual fingerprints). Known as gut microbiota, these bacteria assist with healthy gut function and carry out many important functions, including digesting certain foods, producing vitamins such as vitamin K, folate, and vitamin B_{12}, protecting the intestinal lining by fighting off invaders and forming a barrier effect, and playing an intricate role in the body's immune system.

Part of the role of gut micobiota is to break down undigested food that arrives in the colon, a process called fermentation. Fermentation produces useful by-products, such as short-chain fatty acids. However, it also produces gases. Some gases are absorbed by the blood and excreted through our lungs, while others remain in the gut and pass out of the body in the form of flatulence, often without us even realizing.

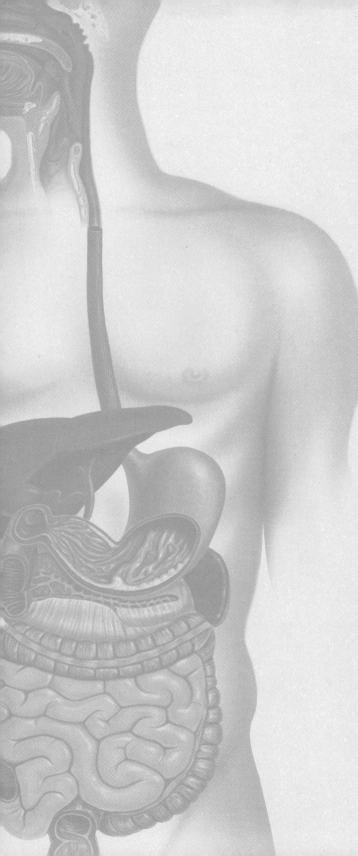

FUNCTIONAL BOWEL DISORDERS

In some people, despite the fact that there is no underlying structural abnormality in the gut, the functioning of the bowel causes abnormal symptoms such as pain, distension, or bloating—so the problem is *functional*, not structural.

Irritable bowel syndrome (IBS) is the name given to a collection of functional bowel symptoms. It is characterized by an altered bowel habit (diarrhea or constipation, or alternating between the two) accompanied by bloating, abdominal pain, or excessive gas. Sufferers may also experience urgency to open their bowels, a need to strain when going to the toilet, feelings of incomplete evacuation after passing a stool, fatigue, "brain fog," and headaches.

The distressing effects of IBS can greatly impact on quality of life. For instance, the symptoms can make it hard for sufferers to even leave the house because of the frequency of necessary trips to the bathroom. The pain can affect enjoyment of life and distract from work. Flatulence causes embarrassment.

Other disorders similar to IBS are functional bloating, functional constipation, and functional pain. Along with IBS, these are collectively known as functional bowel disorders.

Symptoms are often worse after eating and around two-thirds of IBS sufferers perceive diet as being the main factor that influences their symptoms. For this reason they try modifying their diet. Many people embark on a frustrating cycle of restricting food groups without being sure which foods are causing their symptoms. It is common to approach social situations and meals out with trepidation, knowing that, in the majority of the instances, eating in a restaurant will cause a flare-up in symptoms, the causes of which remain a mystery. It is then easy to make the mistake of cutting out the food you think caused the problem when, actually, the cause was something else entirely.

POTENTIAL CAUSES OF FUNCTIONAL BOWEL DISORDERS

The cause of functional bowel disorders is best described as a jigsaw of factors that interplay to cause a symptom profile for each individual. Not all of these factors will play a role in everyone's gut symptoms but it is likely that a number of them will be contributing to your symptoms. Let's look at these pieces of the jigsaw in more detail.

VISCERAL HYPERSENSITIVITY Visceral hypersensitivity, like many areas of functional bowel disorder, is not yet fully understood, but is thought to be affected by a number of factors including genetics, emotional stress, and physical stress (such as a gut infection or gastrointestinal surgery). As described on page 8, the gut is lined with millions of nerve endings that pick up messages from the gut and send them back to the brain. We know people with IBS have super-sensitive nerve endings, which means that the messages sent back to the brain are distorted or hyper-exaggerated, and are often interpreted by the brain as pain. The brain, in turn, "speaks" back to the gut; the way in which the super-sensitive enteric nervous system interprets these messages may result in spasms or changes in motility (the speed of transit and food through the gut).

GUT BACTERIA/MICROFLORA There is increasing evidence that changes or imbalances in our gut bacteria are linked to IBS and other functional gut disorders. We know that people commonly develop gastrointestinal symptoms after a gut infection, such as gastroenteritis or food poisoning, often referred to as post-infectious IBS. At least part of this is thought to be due to changes in the balance of bacteria that live in the gut. People also sometimes experience a flare-up of IBS symptoms after a prolonged or repeated course of antibiotics. Again, this is likely to be due to changes in gut bacteria.

GENETICS Your genes are likely to play an important role in how your gut functions. IBS and digestive issues often run in families—research points to a particular genetic mutation present in IBS suffers. It is likely that specific genes predispose certain people to IBS, and then environmental factors interact with these genes to trigger symptoms.

ANXIETY, DEPRESSION, AND STRESS Research shows there is a strong correlation between anxiety disorders or depression and IBS/gut function. The majority of life stresses are unavoidable, but how we react to stressful situations can be modified. Some people are more prone to anxiety. Interventions that you may want to discuss with your doctor include counseling and psychotherapy, cognitive behavioral therapy, hypnosis, biofeedback therapy (*see opposite*), and medication. Things you can try at home that may help relieve anxiety, reduce stress and enhance your mood are regular exercise, addressing the work-life balance, mindfulness techniques such as yoga and meditation, and finding ways to relax, such as listening to music or taking time each day to get some fresh air.

PHYSICAL STRESS Some people find their gut becomes more sensitive following a physical stressor, such as gastrointestinal or pelvic surgery, gastrointestinal infection, or a period of untreated celiac disease or inflammatory bowel disease (IBD) flare-up.

DIET Diet can impact on IBS symptoms in many ways. As well as FODMAPs, other factors in the diet, such as intake of fiber, fat, resistant starches, and processed foods, can affect digestive symptoms. Your dietitian can discuss how these may be having an impact on you as an individual.

DISTURBED GASTROINTESTINAL MOTILITY Studies suggest that people with IBS sometimes have altered gut motility. Those with diarrhea may have a faster-than-average gut transit time and those with constipation often have slower-than-average transit. It is not yet clear exactly why this change from the norm occurs, but it is likely be a result of messages from the central and enteric nervous system.

COEXISTING CONDITIONS Conditions such as fibromyalgia, endometriosis, and bladder problems can all closely interplay with functional bowel symptoms. Getting the right treatment or taking medication for other health complaints may help ease your gut symptoms.

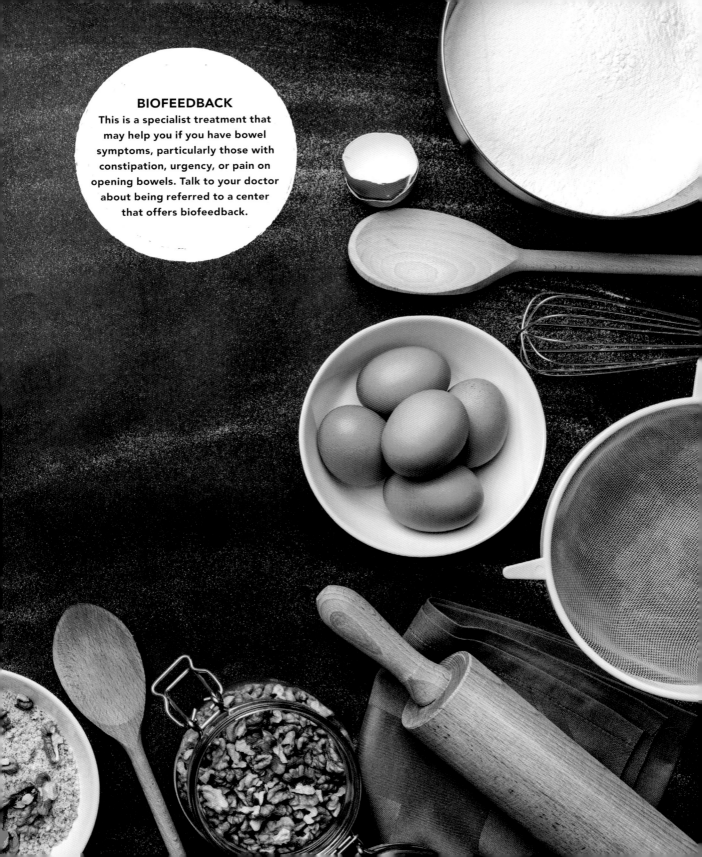

BIOFEEDBACK
This is a specialist treatment that may help you if you have bowel symptoms, particularly those with constipation, urgency, or pain on opening bowels. Talk to your doctor about being referred to a center that offers biofeedback.

HOW A LOW-FODMAP DIET CAN HELP

I have been seeing patients with symptoms of irritable bowel syndrome and digestive distress since 2006. People came to me with a variety of symptom profiles, from bloating and excessive, embarrassing flatulence that affected their confidence, to crippling pain and diarrhea. We would spend time modifying their diets, trialing different exclusions, such as lactose and resistant starches, and adjusting their fiber intake. Often, symptoms improved with dietary changes but, frequently, they didn't improve enough for people to regain their quality of life.

The discovery of the low-FODMAP diet changed my life as a dietitian as well as the lives of thousands of IBS sufferers. Finally, here was a dietary intervention that showed consistent results and improvements in global symptoms. Patients would come back after six to eight weeks on the diet and report that their symptoms had resolved and their lives had changed. Not only does my own clinical practice and that of hundreds of other dietitians reveal that this diet helps, but there are well designed, robust clinical trials that have found that the symptoms of between 65 and 75 percent of IBS sufferers significantly improve or are completely resolved on a low-FODMAP diet.

HOW DO FODMAPS CAUSE SYMPTOMS?

FODMAPs are a group of poorly absorbed fermentable carbohydrates that are present in our diets. Dietitian Sue Shepherd and Gastroenterologist Peter Gibson made a breakthrough in our knowledge of the link between these carbohydrates, diet, and IBS symptoms in the 2000s. They termed the group FODMAPs.

FODMAPs aren't fully digested (broken down) in the gut and therefore can't be completely absorbed. So they remain in the gut, and their presence pulls in more water across the gut wall, which results in a higher volume of intestinal contents, which, in turn, can lead to diarrhea and loose or frequent stools.

As these undigested carbohydrates travel toward and then through the colon, they meet with an increasing number of bacteria (our colonic microflora). These bacteria see the carbohydrate as a readily available food source and ferment them rapidly. This fermentation process produces gas as a byproduct; the volume of gas produced varies from person to person depending on the makeup of their microflora. In susceptible individuals—for example, those with IBS—this gas production can play a significant role in causing symptoms such as abdominal distension (in which the abdominal area becomes larger than normal), bloating (in which the abdominal area *feels* larger than normal), excessive flatulence, abdominal pain, and spasms. It may also contribute to altered gut motility (the speed at which food passes through and is processed in the digestive tract), which can lead to constipation or diarrhea, or often an alternating between the two.

Eliminating these fermentable carbohydrates from the diet or limiting their presence can reduce the volume of gas and liquid in the bowel, thereby improving the symptoms of gastrointestinal distress.

OTHER GUT DISORDERS

The low-FODMAP diet is a useful tool to consider using in the treatment in a variety of other digestive disorders as well as IBS.

INFLAMMATORY BOWEL DISEASE (IBD)

Inflammatory bowel diseases such as Crohn's and ulcerative colitis are autoimmune diseases characterized by intermittent inflammation of the gut wall. The low-FODMAP diet cannot treat the inflammation of the gut that occurs during a flare-up. However, many people with IBD also have a functional bowel disorder such as IBS, and their symptoms exist even when there is no inflammation of the gut wall. At times it is difficult to decipher which gut symptoms are due to a flare-up of IBD, which require medical therapy and which symptoms are due to IBS. This is why, if you have IBD, it's essential that you work with your gastroenterologist and dietitian when deciding whether or not to embark on a low-FODMAP diet.

I have had huge success in using the low-FODMAP diet alongside medical therapy to treat those with IBD. However, it is important to note that people with IBD are more at risk of nutritional depletion, so the involvement of a dietitian is key to success and safety.

CELIAC DISEASE Celiac disease is an autoimmune disease that is characterized by the intolerance to gluten. This is a serious and lifelong condition that must be diagnosed by a doctor. Once diagnosed, the only treatment is a completely gluten-free diet, on which symptoms should improve.

Sometimes, despite sticking rigorously to a gluten-free diet, sufferers of coeliac disease are left with gastrointestinal symptoms, such as bloating and pain, even when their blood results show the disease is under control. These people are likely to have a degree of functional symptoms, possibly as a result of the gut being hypersensitive following a period of damage before the gluten-free diet was undertaken. In this situation the low-FODMAP diet may help address any residual gastrointestinal symptoms.

It's important to realize that while the low-FODMAP diet limits most sources of gluten, it is not a totally gluten-free diet, as it contains limited quantities of gluten-containing grains such as wheat, barley, and rye, and allows gluten in the form of barley malt, oat products, and small amounts of wheat as an ingredient in products such as soy sauce. The celiac sufferer needs to ensure all low-FODMAP products and recipes are checked to avoid even trace amounts of gluten. Another important consideration in celiac disease is calcium intake. Followers of the low-FODMAP diet have been shown to be at risk of not meeting their calcium requirements (see box, right), and as people with celiac disease are at higher risk of low bone density, it is important to take extra care to meet your calcium requirements.

OTHER CAUSES OF DIGESTIVE SYMPTOMS

A low-FODMAP diet may help to treat symptoms of other causes of diarrhea, such as bile acid malabsorption, microscopic colitis, and lymphocytic colitis, by reducing the fermentable carbohydrates in the diet in conjunction with medical treatment offered by your doctor. The low-FODMAP diet may also improve abdominal pain and bloating after gastrointestinal surgery, but be sure to discuss this with your doctor and work with a dietitian.

BEFORE EMBARKING ON A LOW-FODMAP DIET

If you have gastrointestinal symptoms and would like to try the low-FODMAP diet, it is important to first consult your doctor and enlist the help of a dietitian to guide you through the stages of the diet (see page 14). FODMAP intolerances and gastrointestinal symptoms sometimes

CALCIUM

If you are avoiding lactose on the low-FODMAP diet you are at risk of having an inadequate intake of calcium. Some FODMAP-friendly calcium sources are:

- Naturally low-lactose dairy products, such as cheese (see page 16 for more information)

- Lactose-free dairy products, such as lactose-free milk and yogurt

- Calcium-fortified alternative milk and yogurts, such as calcium-enriched almond milk

- Calcium-enriched orange juice (but stick to less than ½ cup per sitting)

- Firm tofu that has been made with calcium sulfate or calcium chloride (note that silken tofu is high FODMAP)

- Fish with small, edible bones, such as smelt (also known in some places as whitebait) or canned salmon

- Kale

feel like a moving target, as there are so many other factors that play a role in combination with diet. For this reason it is important to have guidance from an experienced dietitian.

Your doctor will ask you about the history of your symptoms and carry out screening, including checking for celiac disease (you need to have been eating gluten for the celiac screen to be accurate) and to identify any nutritional deficiencies and how to correct them. Your dietitian will consider your individual symptoms and test results and help you tailor the diet to suit you. He or she can help you get to know the lists of prohibited and limited foods, and also help you find ways in which you can adapt the diet to suit your lifestyle, likes and dislikes, and other dietary restrictions such as veganism, vegetarianism, and coexisting allergies. As you progress through the stages of the diet, your dietitian will be able to troubleshoot for you if you find you are not responding to the diet, help you interpret your response to the diet, and advise you on long-term management of the diet. Crucially, a dietitian can also liaise with your doctor on any medical management of your symptoms alongside dietary management.

FOLLOWING A LOW~FODMAP DIET

The aim of the low-FODMAP diet is to enable you to discover the specific triggers for your individual digestive symptoms. You will discover which FODMAP foods you need to avoid altogether, which you can consume in a limited amount, and which you are able to eat freely. Once you understand how the things you eat affect you, you can establish a tailor-made, long-term modified-FODMAP diet.

The knowledge you gain about which specific foods trigger your symptoms will give you choices by enabling you to weigh up how severe your symptoms will be and how long they will last with how much it suits you to eat that food in a given moment. For example, if you are at a wedding with little choice over the meal you are served and have a relaxing few days ahead in which you can cope with any flare-up of symptoms, you might decide to indulge. On the other hand, you might not want to risk a flare-up and will decide to avoid all your triggers rigorously. The upshot is that the knowledge gives you more control over your diet and symptoms.

THERE ARE THREE STAGES TO THE LOW~FODMAP DIET:

1 THE ELIMINATION PHASE High-FODMAP foods are eliminated.

2 THE RE-CHALLENGE PHASE FODMAPs are reintroduced in a controlled way so you can identify the foods responsible for causing your symptoms.

3 THE MAINTENANCE PHASE You use the knowledge gained during the re-challenge phase to establish a low- or modified-FODMAP diet specific to you.

THE ELIMINATION PHASE

The elimination phase, sometimes called the restriction phase, lasts for four to six weeks. During this time, you discover whether or not your digestive symptoms improve when the quantity of FODMAPs in your system is decreased.

This phase entails avoiding all foods which are high in FODMAPs. Many people notice symptom resolution within a few days. For them, just four weeks is needed for this phase. Those who are a little slower to respond should persevere for six weeks to maximize their chance of seeing their symptoms improve.

People vary in how long they take to respond. Gut transit speed may play a role, and if you tend toward constipation it is likely it will take a bit longer to see symptom response. Fermentable sugars can hang around in the colon for a few days. The aftereffects of the fermentation process and activity of the gut bacteria can affect symptoms for longer than a few days. It has been suggested in one study that symptoms can occur for up to 30 days after ingestion of FODMAPs. For this reason you will get the best, most consistent response if you are as strict as possible regarding your intake of FODMAPs during the elimination phase. It is worth persevering. I have had clients who have not improved until week five, then have had the most miraculous change in their symptoms.

All five FODMAP groups must be avoided initially, because it is common to have a problematic response to more than one FODMAP family. Cutting them out one at a time often won't lead to significant symptom improvement because other FODMAPs that may be causing symptoms will still be present in the diet. (There are exceptions to this rule when it comes to fructose and lactose. *See* the information on page 16, and ask your dietitian for further advice.)

It is virtually impossible to cut out all FODMAPs present in the diet—that is why we call this the low-FODMAP diet, not the no-FODMAP diet. However, try your best to avoid all the foods that are high in FODMAPs. It is important to be as consistent as possible in the elimination phase.

HOW TO AVOID FODMAPS

The table opposite lists the foods that are restricted on a low-FODMAP diet. This is not an exhaustive list, since the understanding of the FODMAP content of foods is developing all the time. Your dietitian will provide you with the most up-to-date information on portion sizes and foods you can include or should avoid. Many foods contain more than one type of FODMAP, for instance cashews and pistachios contain both fructans and galacto-oligosaccharides. For the re-introduction process you will need more information from your dietitian on how the groups overlap between foods.

What to AVOID
and what to LIMIT

FOOD	AVOID		ALLOW IN SMALL AMOUNTS	
VEGETABLES	• Asparagus • Beans (apart from green snap beans) • Belgian endive root • Cauliflower • Edamame beans • Garlic (including garlic puree, garlic salt, garlic powder, garlic flavoring—unless strained garlic oil) • Jerusalem artichoke • Leeks	• Mushrooms • Onions (including onion salt, onion flavoring, onion powder) • Sugar snap peas • White part of scallion	• Avocado • Beets • Broccoli • Brussels sprouts • Butternut squash • Cassava • Celery • Corn • Fennel bulb • Globe artichoke • Lentils • Snow peas • Okra	• Peas • Savoy cabbage • Sweet potato
FRUITS	• Apples • Blackberries • Cherries • Figs • Goji berries • Mangoes • Pears • Stone fruits: peaches,	nectarines, apricots, plums, prunes, dates • Watermelon	• Coconut • Grapefruit • Lychees • Pomegranate • Tamarind • Limit all other fruit to 1 portion per sitting	
STARCHY FOODS	• Amaranth • Barley • Flours, breads, cakes, pasta made from the above grains • Rye	• Spelt flakes • Spelt pasta • Wheat (trace amounts are allowed, such as that in soy sauce)		
ADDED INGREDIENTS	• Agave nectar • FOS (fructo-oligosaccharide) • Fructose • Fructose-glucose syrup, fructose corn syrup, high-fructose	corn syrup • Honey • Inulin • Oligofructose • Prebiotics • Sorbitol, xylitol and mannitol		
DRINKS	• Avoid all fruit juice from non-allowed fruit • Chamomile tea • Chicory root tea • Coconut water • Dandelion tea	• Dessert wine • Fennel tea • Oolang tea • Rum	• No more than ½ cup fruit juice	
NUTS	• Cashews • Pistachios		• All other nuts and seeds limit to a handful per sitting	
DAIRY PRODUCTS	• *See* box on lactose intolerance on page 16			

FRUCTOSE INTOLERANCE Around 40 percent of people don't absorb fructose, leading to digestive symptoms. It is difficult to know if you are in that 40 percent. I usually recommend that people avoid fructose in the elimination phase so all bases are covered. Ask your dietitian for advice—you may have the option of being referred for a fructose breath test by your healthcare professional to determine whether or not you are malabsorbing fructose. The best way to diagnose fructose intolerance is to avoid fructose for a period of four to six weeks, then reintroduce it and monitor symptoms.

LACTOSE INTOLERANCE Around 5 percent of people of Northern European descent malabasorb lactose. The prevalence is higher in those of Southern European descent, and is even higher in those of Asian or African descent. If this malabsorbed lactose goes on to cause symptoms, this is called lactose intolerance (not everyone who malabsorbs lactose experiences symptoms). A lactose breath test can be helpful to determine lactose malabsorption, but the results need to be interpreted by someone with expertise in this area. As with fructose, the most accurate way to tell if you have a lactose intolerance is to cut out

LACTOSE
what to AVOID and what to CHOOSE

AVOID ON A LOW-LACTOSE DIET	SUITABLE CHOICES FOR A LOW-LACTOSE/LOW-FODMAP DIET
• All animal milks including cow, goat, and sheep (unless it is specifically labeled as lactose-free)	• Plant milks such as almond, hemp, oat, and rice • Small portions of coconut milk (less than ¼ cup) • Soy milk in limited quantities** • Specifically lactose-free milk milk (whole, semiskim, skim)
• Yogurt	• Coconut-based yogurts (most on the market contain hidden FODMAPs but new brands are appearing all the time so keep your eye out and read the ingredients thoroughly). It is not clear what the maximum portion size of coconut yogurt is to ensure it is still low FODMAP so exercise caution and stick to small amounts, less than 3 tablespoons per sitting, and monitor tolerance. • Lactose-free yogurts (fruit or plain) • Soy yogurts ** • *It is important to check ingredients and avoid FODMAP fruits, added fructose, xylitol, inulin, or FOS*
• Cottage cheese, cream cheese, halloumi, low-fat cheese, processed cheeses such as cheese strings and cheese slices, quark, ricotta	• Most other cheese including ripened cheeses like Brie and Camembert
• Custard • Ice cream	• Butter • Cream • Crème fraîche • Dark chocolate, small portions of milk chocolate • Sour cream • Soy custard and soy ice cream** • *You do not need to use special lactose-free butters, cream, and hard cheese*

sources of lactose completely for at least four weeks, then reintroduce it using foods containing increasing amounts of lactose over a three-day period. This is often most successful when done alongside the restriction of other FODMAPs.

The recipes in this book are all suitable for a low-lactose diet (including the elimination phase of the low-FODMAP diet). However, if you know that you tolerate lactose well, you can use normal milk and yogurt instead of lactose-free or plant-based alternatives in the recipes, as long as you check the products you select for other FODMAP ingredients, such as FODMAP fruits or added fructose.

Most people with lactose intolerance can usually tolerate small amounts of lactose and that is why I recommend a low-lactose diet rather than a lactose-free diet. The table opposite gives guidance on what you need to limit to follow a low-lactose diet.

THOSE PESKY LABELS

You will need to check the labels of any packaged foods you eat carefully to ensure they don't contain foods listed in the avoid columns on pages 15 and 17. There are several low-FODMAP apps that can help with this (*see Resources, page 224*). I would recommend choosing one that is based on foods available where you live, such as the Monash University Low FODMAP Diet app, which can be used in conjunction with your dietitian.

← ***Soy milk contains galacto-oligosaccharides and, although suitable for a low-lactose diet, should be restricted to ¼ cup per serving on the low-FODMAP diet. It is not currently clear how much of these galacto-oligosaccharides are found in soy yogurt and soy ice cream, but they are likely to be similar to soy milk and, for this reason, I would proceed with caution and limit to small portions only i.e. 2 tablespoons.*

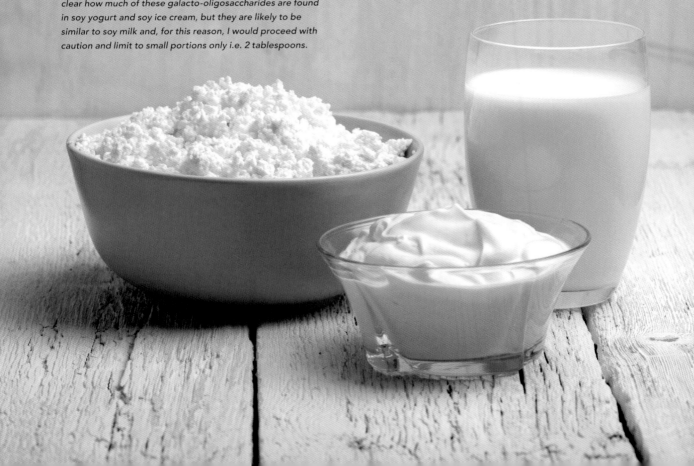

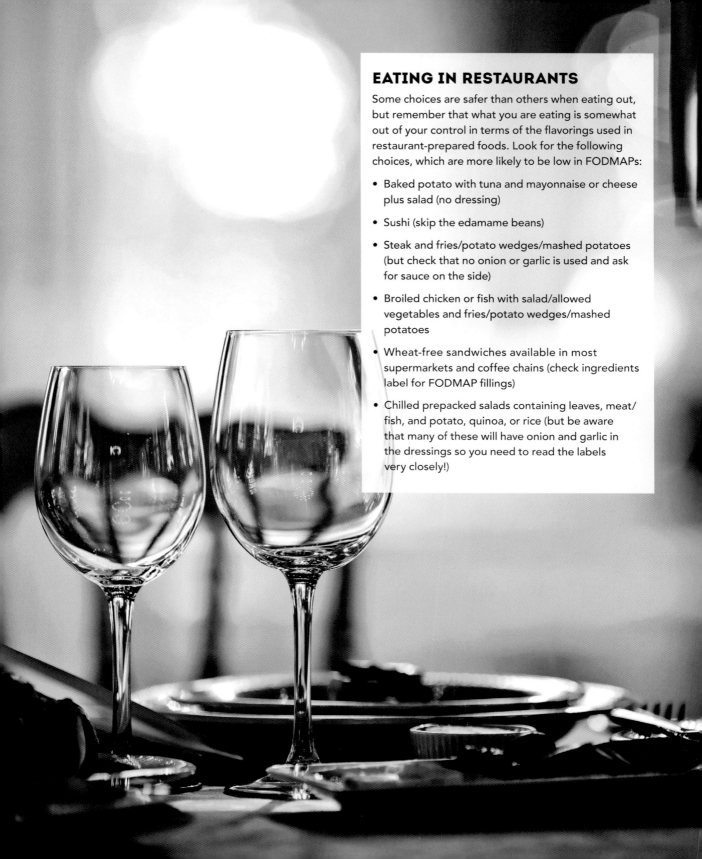

EATING IN RESTAURANTS

Some choices are safer than others when eating out, but remember that what you are eating is somewhat out of your control in terms of the flavorings used in restaurant-prepared foods. Look for the following choices, which are more likely to be low in FODMAPs:

• Baked potato with tuna and mayonnaise or cheese plus salad (no dressing)

• Sushi (skip the edamame beans)

• Steak and fries/potato wedges/mashed potatoes (but check that no onion or garlic is used and ask for sauce on the side)

• Broiled chicken or fish with salad/allowed vegetables and fries/potato wedges/mashed potatoes

• Wheat-free sandwiches available in most supermarkets and coffee chains (check ingredients label for FODMAP fillings)

• Chilled prepacked salads containing leaves, meat/fish, and potato, quinoa, or rice (but be aware that many of these will have onion and garlic in the dressings so you need to read the labels very closely!)

WHY HAVEN'T I RESPONDED?

Some IBS sufferers do not get adequate relief from their IBS on the low-FODMAP diet. So why aren't you responding?

UNKNOWN FODMAPS SNEAKING INTO YOUR DIET Schedule a review with your dietitian to go through your diet to look for hidden suspects. If you don't have regular access to a dietitian you might find that keeping a food and symptom diary for one to two weeks, then looking back on it, can help identify if you have slipped up. Symptoms can last for between a few hours to a few weeks. So if you are slipping up weekly it could appear you are not responding to the low-FODMAP diet when, in fact, the failure to improve is due to not sticking to the diet. Remember to check ingredients on labels of anything prepackaged. Especially beware of "flavorings" that may contain onion or garlic powder and "sweeteners" that may contain any of the polyols. Are you eating in restaurants a lot? To get the best out of the elimination phase, be discerning about how frequently and where you eat out during these few weeks, as hidden FODMAPs in restaurant food may be a contributor to not responding fully to the diet. Also, check your medication and supplements for hidden FODMAPs such as inulin, FOS, and sorbitol.

EATING LARGE QUANTITIES OF THE "FOODS TO BE EATEN IN MODERATION" There are a number of foods that are allowed on the low-FODMAP diet if eaten in moderation. But if you consume too much of these foods you give your body a high-FODMAP load, so it's important to stick to the portion sizes suggested by your dietitian. You may find using the FoodMaestro FODMAP app (created by the low-FODMAP team at King's College London) in conjunction with information provided by your dietitian helpful in determining safe portions.

EATING TOO MUCH FRUIT IN ONE SITTING Even low-FODMAP fruit can cause digestive symptoms if you consume more than 2¾ oz during one sitting. The same is true for fruit juice. Limit fruit juices allowed on the diet to ½ cup per sitting.

NON-DIETARY FACTORS ARE AFFECTING YOUR SYMPTOMS Two of the most common culprits for not getting adequate relief of your symptoms on the low-FODMAP diet are stress and anxiety. One scenario I often encounter is a client initially doing well in terms of symptom response on the diet, who then encounters a stressful week at work or family stress and sees their symptoms immediately multiply.

CONSTIPATION Sometimes people become constipated on the low-FODMAP diet and need to take extra steps to ensure good gut motility. Being constipated is likely to cause abdominal discomfort even if you are avoiding FODMAPs, so enlist your doctor's or dietitian's help to address this issue alongside doing the diet.

UNDERLYING PROBLEMS WITH GASTROINTESTINAL TRACT It is important to involve your doctor and dietitian from the beginning when starting on a low-FODMAP diet so they can rule out other disorders such as celiac disease, inflammatory bowel disease, small intestinal bacteria overgrowth (SIBO), bile acid malabsorption, microscopic colitis, and so on.

THE RE-CHALLENGE AND MAINTENANCE PHASES

Once you feel your symptoms have adequately improved after the elimination phase, your dietitian will take you through the re-challenge or reintroduction phase in a structured manner. In this phase you start re-challenging your gut with higher-FODMAP foods by systematically introducing them, with the aim of identifying which FODMAP families cause your symptoms and how much of them you can consume before experiencing symptoms. This information is called your individual threshold level. If you need further information alongside your dietitian's advice, I recommend the book by Lee Martin RD on FODMAP re-challenge and reintroduction mentioned in the Resources section (*see* page 224).

Once you have established your individual threshold levels, your dietitian will help you to embark on the third phase of the FODMAP diet, the maintenance phase, which is often referred to as the modified-FODMAP diet.

A FINAL WORD

The recipes in this book have been checked to ensure that the portion sizes are "safe" within the limitations of the ingredients, so it is important to follow the "serves" information to prevent you from consuming too many FODMAPs.

BREAKFAST & BRUNCH

CONSUMING
1 TABLESPOON OF
FLAXSEEDS PER DAY
IS AN EFFECTIVE WAY OF
PREVENTING CONSTIPATION.
ENSURE YOU TAKE THEM WITH
A LARGE GLASS OF WATER,
TO HELP THE FLAXSEEDS
DO THEIR JOB.

PREPARATION TIME: 5 MINUTES
COOKING TIME: 25 TO 30 MINUTES
SERVES: 2

$2\frac{1}{2}$ cups lactose-free or plant-based milk (limit soy to $\frac{1}{4}$ cup per portion), or standard milk if you know you tolerate lactose

$\frac{1}{2}$ cup quinoa

$\frac{1}{2}$ teaspoon ground cinnamon

1 cup fresh raspberries

2 tablespoons mixed seeds (such as sunflower seeds, flaxseeds, pumpkin seeds, and hemp seeds)

1 to 2 tablespoons maple syrup, to taste

QUINOA PORRIDGE
WITH RASPBERRIES

Bring the milk to a boil in a small saucepan. Add the quinoa and return to boiling. Reduce the heat to low, cover the pan with a lid, and let simmer for about 15 minutes, until three-quarters of the milk has been absorbed.

Stir the cinnamon into the pan, cover, and cook for 8 to 10 minutes or until almost all the milk has been absorbed and the quinoa is tender.

Spoon the porridge into 2 bowls, top with the raspberries, sprinkle with the seeds, and drizzle with the maple syrup. Serve immediately.

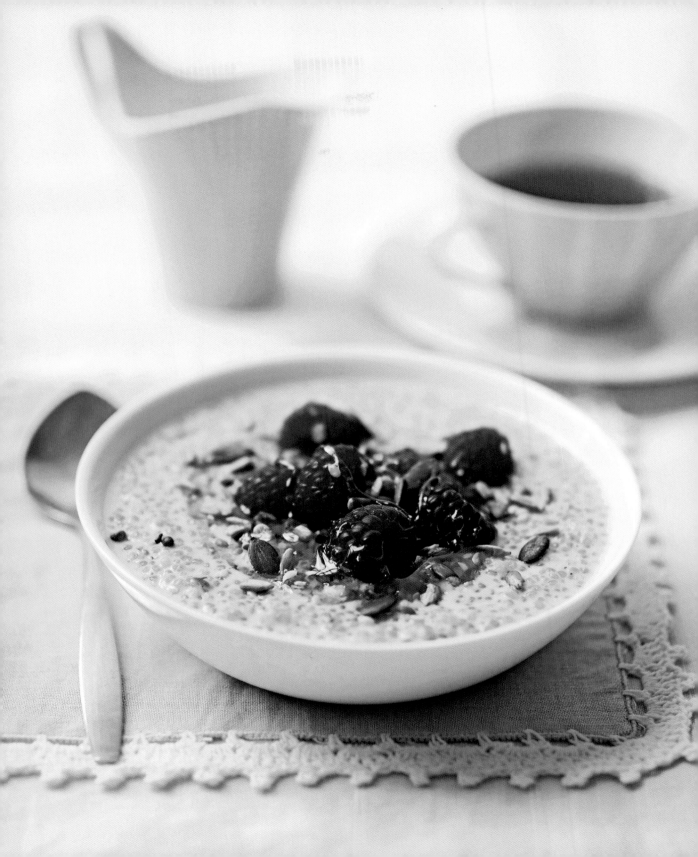

spray olive oil, for greasing

2 cups rolled oats

2³⁄₄oz mixed low-FODMAP nuts (such as peanuts, walnuts, and macadamia nuts), toasted and coarsely chopped

1 tablespoon maple syrup, plus extra to serve

1¼ cups lactose-free or plant-based milk (limit soy to ¼ cup per portion), or standard milk if you know you tolerate lactose, plus extra to serve

1 cup mixed low-FODMAP summer berries (such as raspberries and strawberries)

plain lactose-free or plant-based yogurt (limit soy yogurt to ¼ cup), or standard yogurt if you know you tolerate lactose

NOT ONLY ARE OATS HELPFUL FOR RELIEVING CONSTIPATION, THE SOLUBLE FIBER THEY CONTAIN HELPS TO LOWER CHOLESTEROL AND STABILIZE BLOOD SUGARS, HELPING TO KEEP YOU FULL UNTIL LUNCHTIME.

SUMMER BERRY GRANOLA

PREPARATION TIME: 10 MINUTES, PLUS COOLING
COOKING TIME: 10 MINUTES
SERVES: 4

Preheat the oven to 350°F. Spray a baking pan lightly with spray oil.

Add the oats and nuts to a bowl and stir in the maple syrup. Spread the mixture evenly onto the prepared baking sheet, place in the oven, and bake for 5 minutes.

Remove the mixture from the oven and stir well. Return to the oven and bake for a further 3 to 4 minutes, until lightly toasted. Let cool.

Divide the granola between 4 serving bowls and add the milk. Scatter with the berries and serve with yogurt and a drizzle of maple syrup.

BIRCHER MUESLI

PREPARATION TIME: 10 MINUTES

SERVES: 4

2 cups rolled oats

3½oz mixed low-FODMAP nuts
(such as peanuts, walnuts, and
macadamia nuts), toasted and
coarsely chopped

1 tablespoon maple syrup,
plus extra to serve

2½ cups lactose-free
or plant-based milk (limit
soy to ¼ cup per portion),
or standard milk if you know
you tolerate lactose, plus
extra to serve

1 cup mixed low-FODMAP summer
berries (such as raspberries
and strawberries)

plain lactose-free or
plant-based yogurt (limit
soy yogurt to ¼ cup per
portion), or standard yogurt
if you know you tolerate
lactose, to serve (optional)

Add the oats and nuts to a bowl, stir in the maple syrup, and then stir in the milk. Let the mixture soak for at least 2 hours or overnight in the refrigerator.

Divide the muesli between 4 bowls and serve topped with the mixed berries and yogurt, if using, with extra maple syrup for drizzling.

2 cups rolled oats

2 lactose-free or plant-based milk (limit soy to $\frac{1}{4}$ cup per portion), or standard milk if you know you tolerate lactose

$2\frac{1}{2}$ cups water

3 tablespoons freshly grated coconut

$\frac{1}{4}$ cup plain lactose-free or plant-based yogurt (limit soy yogurt to $\frac{1}{4}$ cup per portion), or standard yogurt if you know you tolerate lactose

$1\frac{1}{3}$ cups fresh berries (such as raspberries, blueberries, and hulled strawberries)

$\frac{1}{4}$ cup maple syrup (optional)

REMEMBER WHEN USING COCONUT TO LIMIT FRESH COCONUT TO 3 TABLESPOONS PER PORTION, AND DESICCATED COCONUT TO 1 TABLESPOON PER PORTION.

BERRY & COCONUT PORRIDGE

PREPARATION TIME: 5 MINUTES
COOKING TIME: 10 MINUTES
SERVES: 4

Put the oats into a saucepan with the milk and measured water. Bring to a boil, then simmer for 8 minutes, stirring often, until thick and creamy.

Pour the porridge into 4 warmed bowls. Divide the grated coconut and yogurt between the bowls and stir them into the porridge. Scatter with the berries and drizzle with maple syrup, if using, and serve immediately.

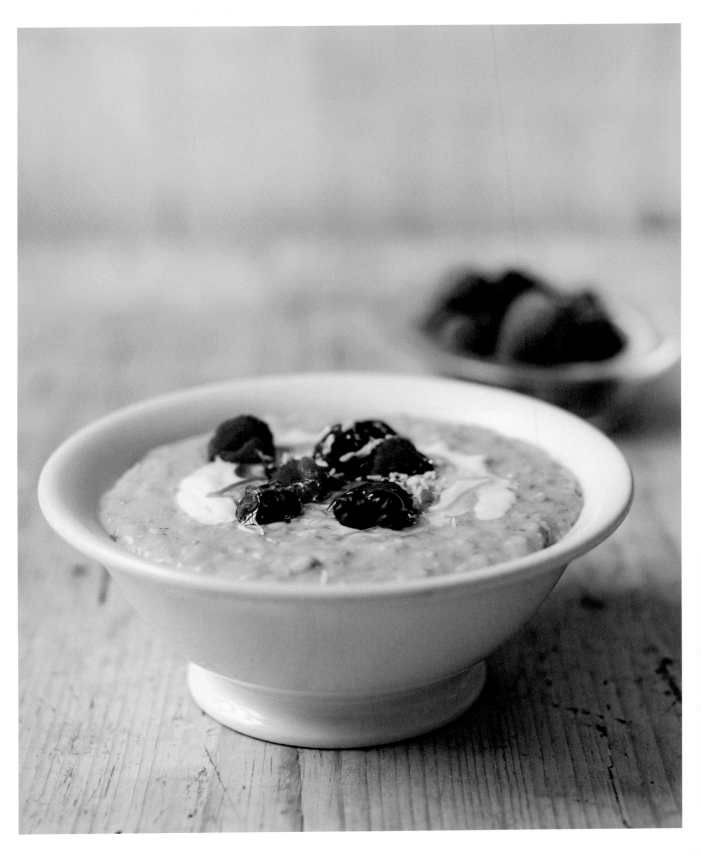

CUCUMBER, LEMON & MINT SMOOTHIE

PREPARATION TIME: 5 MINUTES
SERVES: 3

9oz cucumber, peeled and
coarsely chopped
....
2 tablespoons lemon juice
....
3 to 4 mint leaves
....
2 to 3 ice cubes
....
strips of cucumber, to
decorate (optional)

Put the cucumber, lemon juice, mint leaves, and ice cubes into a blender or the bowl of a food processor and process briefly.

Pour the smoothie into 3 tall glasses, decorate each with a strip of cucumber, if liked, and serve immediately.

1 ripe banana

....

1¼ cups lactose-free or plant-based milk (limit soy milk to ¼ cup per portion), or standard milk if you know you tolerate lactose

....

1 tablespoon smooth peanut butter (free from high-fructose corn syrup)

PEANUT BUTTER IS A FANTASTIC SOURCE OF PROTEIN AND CALORIES, WHICH CAN BE ESPECIALLY HELPFUL IF YOU ARE STRUGGLING TO MAINTAIN YOUR WEIGHT ON THE LOW-FODMAP DIET.

BANANA & PEANUT BUTTER SMOOTHIE

PREPARATION TIME: 5 MINUTES, PLUS 2 HOURS FREEZING

SERVES: 1

Peel the banana and cut it into slices. Transfer the slices to a freezerproof container and freeze for at least 2 hours or overnight.

Put the frozen banana, milk, and peanut butter into a blender or the bowl of a food processor and process until smooth.

Pour the smoothie into a tall glass and serve immediately.

2 eggs, beaten

1 teaspoon vanilla extract

½ cup lactose-free or plant-based milk (limit soy milk to ¼ cup per portion), or standard milk if you know you tolerate lactose

1 tablespoon superfine sugar

½ teaspoon ground cinnamon

8 slices of gluten-free bread

2 tablespoons butter

confectioners' sugar, for dusting

fruit, to serve (optional)

IF YOU WANT TO SERVE THESE WITH FRUIT, BE CAREFUL NOT TO OVERDOSE ON IT. AIM FOR A MAXIMUM OF 2¾ OZ TOTAL FRUIT PER SERVING TO ENSURE EACH MEAL REMAINS LOW FODMAP.

FRENCH TOAST

PREPARATION TIME: 5 MINUTES
COOKING TIME: 5 MINUTES
SERVES: 4

Beat together the eggs, vanilla extract, milk, sugar, and cinnamon in a shallow dish. Place the slices of bread in the mixture, turning them over to coat both sides and so that they absorb the liquid.

Heat the butter in a nonstick skillet over medium heat. Use a metal spatula or a lifter to remove the soaked bread from the dish and fry the slices for 2 minutes on each side, or until golden. Cut the toast in half diagonally into triangles, dust with a little confectioners' sugar, and serve immediately.

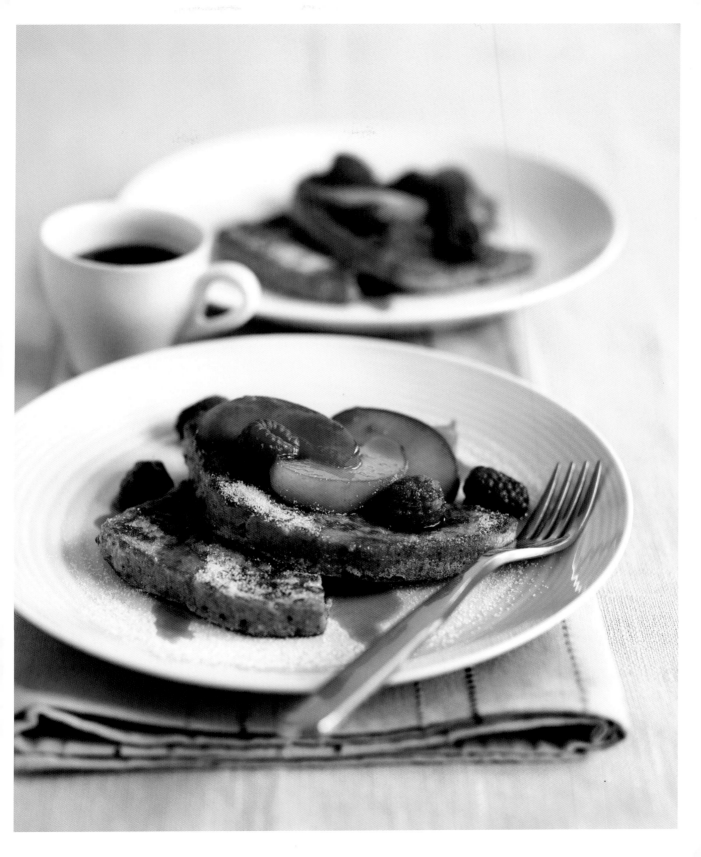

PREPARATION TIME: 15 MINUTES,
    PLUS PROVING AND COOLING
COOKING TIME: ABOUT 40
    MINUTES
MAKES: 1 LOAF

3¾ cups buckwheat flour, plus extra for dusting

3 tablespoons ground flaxseeds

1 teaspoon salt

1 teaspoon sugar

⅓ cup psyllium husk powder

3 tablespoons pumpkin seeds, divided

2½ cups warm water

2½ teaspoons active dry yeast

2 tablespoons coconut or olive oil, plus extra for brushing

GLUTEN-FREE BUCKWHEAT BREAD

In a large bowl, mix together the buckwheat flour, ground flaxseeds, salt, sugar, psyllium husk powder, and 2 tablespoons of the pumpkin seeds. In a large measuring cup, whisk the water with the yeast.

Pour the yeast mixture and oil into the flour mixture and mix well to make a sticky dough.

Tip out the dough onto a lightly floured surface and knead lightly for about 10 seconds, then return the dough to the bowl, cover the bowl with plastic wrap, and let stand in a warm place for 30 minutes to rise.

Line a cookie sheet with nonstick parchment paper.

Shape the dough into a fat sausage, then brush it with oil and scatter with the remaining pumpkin seeds. Transfer the dough to the prepared cookie sheet, cover the dough with a clean dish cloth, and let rise in a warm place for 30 minutes.

Preheat the oven to 425°F.

Uncover the dough. Slash the top several times with a sharp knife and dust with a little buckwheat flour. Bake for 35 to 40 minutes, or until the loaf is golden brown and sounds hollow when tapped on the bottom. Let cool on a wire rack before slicing.

PREPARATION TIME: 25
   MINUTES, PLUS 4 DAYS
   STARTER FERMENTATION,
   APPROXIMATELY 18 HOURS
   PROVING, AND COOLING
COOKING TIME: 40 TO 45 MINUTES
MAKES: 1 LARGE LOAF

FOR THE STARTER

2½ cups stoneground
wholegrain spelt flour, divided

1½ cups tepid water, divided

FOR THE BREAD

1¾ cups warm water

2 teaspoons sugar

¾ cup starter (see left)

4¼ cups wholegrain spelt
flour, plus extra for dusting

2 teaspoons salt

ALTHOUGH
SPELT PASTA, SPELT
FLAKES, AND STANDARD
SPELT BREADS ARE NOT
PERMISSIBLE ON THE
LOW-FODMAP DIET,
100 PERCENT SOURDOUGH
SPELT BREAD IS. WHY NOT
TRY MAKING YOUR
OWN?

SPELT SOURDOUGH LOAF

To make the starter, put one-third of the flour into a plastic container. Add one-third of the measured water. Stir well to make a paste. Cover and let stand for 48 hours.

After this time, small bubbles should have appeared on the surface. Stir in another third of the flour and third of the water. Repeat this process 24 hours later using the remaining flour and water. By day 4, your starter should be ready—it will be frothy, will have large bubbles.

To make the bread, mix the warm water and sugar in a large bowl, then stir in the starter until well blended. Mix in the flour and salt to make a sticky dough. Cover the bowl loosely with plastic wrap or a clean dish cloth and let prove for 1 hour.

With lightly floured hands, stretch and fold the dough in the bowl, cover loosely, and let prove for 30 minutes. Repeat this process twice more, then cover loosely and let rise overnight or for about 6 hours, until the dough has doubled in volume.

Tip the dough onto a floured surface and shape it into a round loaf. Place it in a silicone breadmaker or a preheated Dutch oven (if you bake it on a cookie sheet, the loaf will spread out too much). Let prove for a further 30 to 40 minutes.

Preheat the oven to 425°F.

Dust the top of the dough with a little flour and make 2 slashes in the top. Bake for 40 to 45 minutes, until the loaf is golden brown and sounds hollow when tapped on the bottom. If cooking it in a Dutch oven, remove the lid for the last 10 minutes of cooking. Transfer the loaf to a wire rack to cool, then slice.

(You will have some starter left over after following this recipe, which you can use to make more bread if you keep it alive. To do so, continue to feed it by stirring in flour and water once a week, and store it in the refrigerator loosely covered.)

1 cup gluten-free
self-rising flour

1 teaspoon gluten-free
baking powder

1 egg

$\frac{2}{3}$ cup lactose-free or plant-based milk (limit soy to
$\frac{1}{4}$ cup per portion), or
standard milk if you know
you tolerate lactose

2 tablespoons unsalted butter,
margarine, or coconut oil,
melted

$\frac{2}{3}$ cup blueberries, divided

1 tablespoon olive oil

TO SERVE

plain or fruit lactose-free or
plant-based yogurt (limit soy
yogurt to $\frac{1}{4}$ cup per portion),
or standard yogurt if you
know you tolerate lactose

maple syrup (optional)

BLUEBERRY PANCAKES
WITH YOGURT

PREPARATION TIME: 10 MINUTES
COOKING TIME: 20 MINUTES
SERVES: 4

Mix together the flour and baking powder in a large bowl.

Beat together the egg and milk in a large measuring cup. Pour the wet mixture into the flour and beat until smooth.

Beat in the melted butter, margarine, or coconut oil, then gently stir in half of the blueberries.

Heat the oil in a nonstick skillet over medium heat. Spoon the batter a tablespoonful at a time into the skillet. Cook for 3 to 4 minutes until golden on the underside, then flip the pancakes over and cook for a further 2 to 3 minutes. Repeat with the remaining batter.

Serve with the remaining blueberries, a dollop of yogurt, and a drizzle of maple syrup, if using.

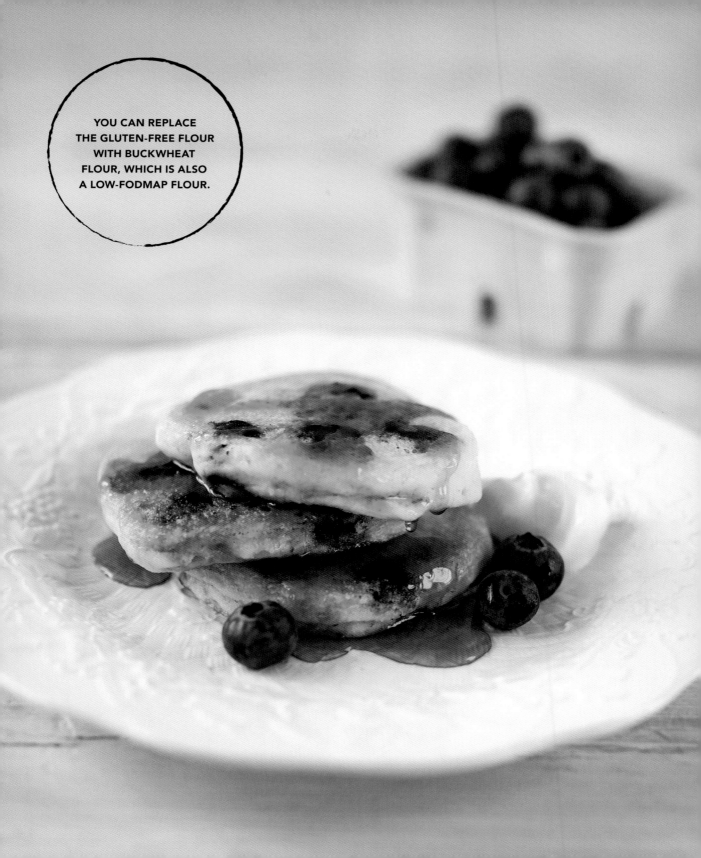

YOU CAN REPLACE
THE GLUTEN-FREE FLOUR
WITH BUCKWHEAT
FLOUR, WHICH IS ALSO
A LOW-FODMAP FLOUR.

- 1¼ cups gluten-free all-purpose flour
- 1¼ cups gluten-free self-rising flour
- 1 tablespoon baking powder
- ¼ cup packed light brown sugar
- 3 pieces of stem ginger in syrup from a jar (about 1¾oz), finely chopped
- ⅔ cup frozen or fresh blueberries
- 1 egg
- 1 cup lactose-free or plant-based milk (limit soy to ¼ cup per portion), or standard milk if you know you tolerate lactose
- ¼ cup vegetable oil

THESE MAKE A GREAT ON-THE-GO SNACK OR BREAKFAST, AND FREEZE WELL TOO. JUST DEFROST ONE OVERNIGHT AND SLING IT IN YOUR BAG AS YOU ARE RUNNING OUT THE DOOR.

BLUEBERRY & GINGER MUFFINS

PREPARATION TIME: 10 MINUTES, PLUS COOLING
COOKING TIME: 20 MINUTES
SERVES: 12

Preheat the oven to 400°F. Line a 12-hole muffin pan with paper muffin cups.

Sift the flours and baking powder into a large bowl. Stir in the sugar, ginger, and blueberries until they are evenly distributed.

Beat together the egg, milk, and oil in a large measuring cup, then add the liquid to the flour mixture. Using a large metal spoon, gently stir the liquid into the flour until only just combined. The batter should look craggy, with specks of flour still visible.

Divide the batter between the muffin cups, piling it up in the center of each cup. Bake for 18 to 20 minutes, until well risen and golden. Transfer to a wire rack and let cool a little. Serve while still slightly warm.

BREAKFAST CEREAL BARS

PREPARATION TIME: 10 MINUTES
COOKING TIME: 35 MINUTES
MAKES: 16

1 stick softened butter or ½ cup coconut oil, plus extra for greasing

3 tablespoons soft light brown sugar

2 tablespoons corn syrup

½ cup millet flakes

¼ cup quinoa

½ cup dried cranberries

½ cup blanched peanuts

¼ cup sunflower seeds

2½ tablespoons sesame seeds

2½ tablespoons flaxseeds

½ cup unsweetened desiccated coconut

Preheat the oven to 350°F. Grease an 11 x 8 inch shallow baking pan.

Beat together the butter or coconut oil, sugar, and syrup in a large bowl until creamy. Add the remaining ingredients and beat well until combined.

Spoon the mixture into the prepared pan and level off the surface with the back of a spoon. Bake for 35 minutes, until deep golden. Remove the pan from the oven and let the cereal block cool in the pan.

Turn out the block onto a wooden cutting board and carefully slice it into 16 fingers using a serrated knife. Store in an airtight container for up to 5 days.

4 zucchini, grated

¼ cup gluten-free
self-rising flour

½ cup Parmesan cheese, grated

2 tablespoons olive oil

4 eggs

freshly ground black pepper

ZUCCHINI FRITTERS
WITH POACHED EGGS

PREPARATION TIME: 10 MINUTES
COOKING TIME: 20 MINUTES
SERVES: 4

Place the grated zucchini, flour, and grated Parmesan in a bowl and mix together well. Squeeze chunks of the mixture into walnut-sized balls and then gently flatten them into patties.

Heat the oil in a deep skillet and, working in batches if necessary, fry the fritters for 2 to 3 minutes on each side, until golden.

Meanwhile, bring a large saucepan of water to a gentle simmer and stir with a large spoon to create a swirl. Carefully break 2 eggs into the water and cook for 3 minutes. Remove the eggs with a slotted spoon and keep warm. Repeat with the remaining eggs.

Serve the fritters topped with the poached eggs and sprinkled with black pepper.

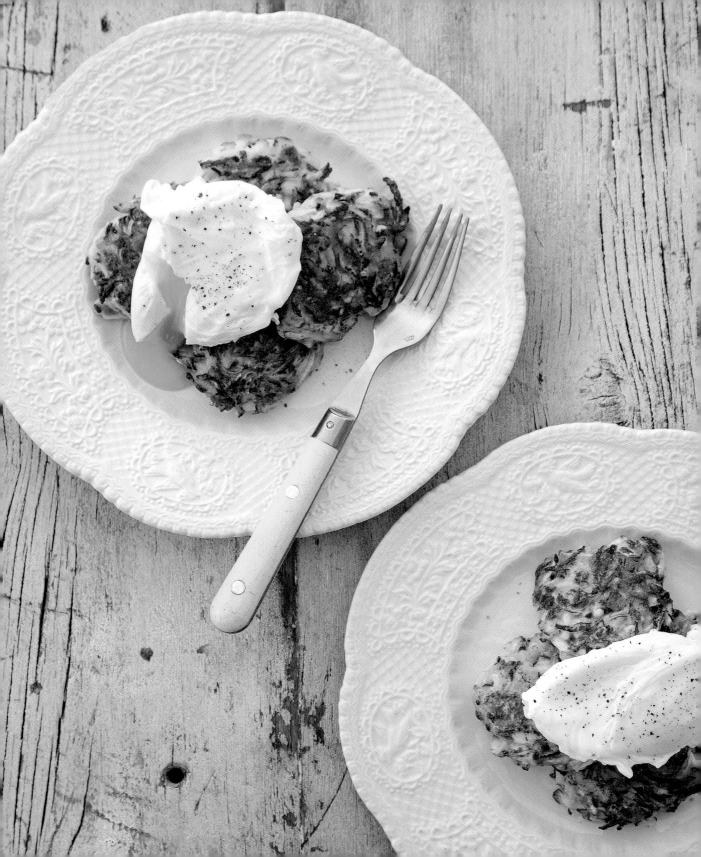

1 tablespoon butter or olive
oil

.....

1lb spinach

pinch of grated nutmeg

4 large eggs

grated Cheddar cheese,
for sprinkling

salt and freshly ground
black pepper

FOR THE CHEESE SAUCE

1½ tablespoons butter

2½ tablespoons gluten-free
all-purpose flour

¼ teaspoon English mustard

1¼ cups lactose-free or
plant-based milk (limit soy
to ¼ cup per portion), or
standard milk if you know
you tolerate lactose

½ cup sharp Cheddar cheese,
grated

IT IS A COMMON
MISCONCEPTION THAT
ALL DAIRY PRODUCTS
SHOULD BE AVOIDED ON A
LOW-FODMAP DIET. CHEDDAR,
AND MANY OTHER CHEESES,
ARE LOW IN LACTOSE AND,
THEREFORE, SUITABLE
IN MODERATION.

EGGS FLORENTINE

PREPARATION TIME: 5 MINUTES
COOKING TIME: 20 MINUTES
SERVES: 4

Preheat the broiler on the highest setting.

First make the cheese sauce. Melt the butter in a small saucepan over low heat, then stir in the flour and mustard. Cook, stirring continuously, for 1 minute.

Pour in the milk gradually, whisking to remove any lumps, then cook over low heat, stirring continuously, until the mixture begins to boil. Reduce the heat to simmer, then stir in two-thirds of the Cheddar.

Meanwhile, melt the butter or heat the oil in a saucepan, add the spinach, and cook over medium heat for 3 to 4 minutes, until the spinach has wilted. Season with salt and pepper, then stir in the nutmeg. Transfer the mixture to an ovenproof dish or divide it between 4 individual ovenproof dishes.

Poach the eggs in a deep skillet of simmering water for 4 to 5 minutes, then drain and place them on top of the spinach. Pour the cheese sauce over the eggs and sprinkle with the grated Cheddar. Place the dish or dishes under the hot broiler and cook until golden and bubbling. Serve immediately.

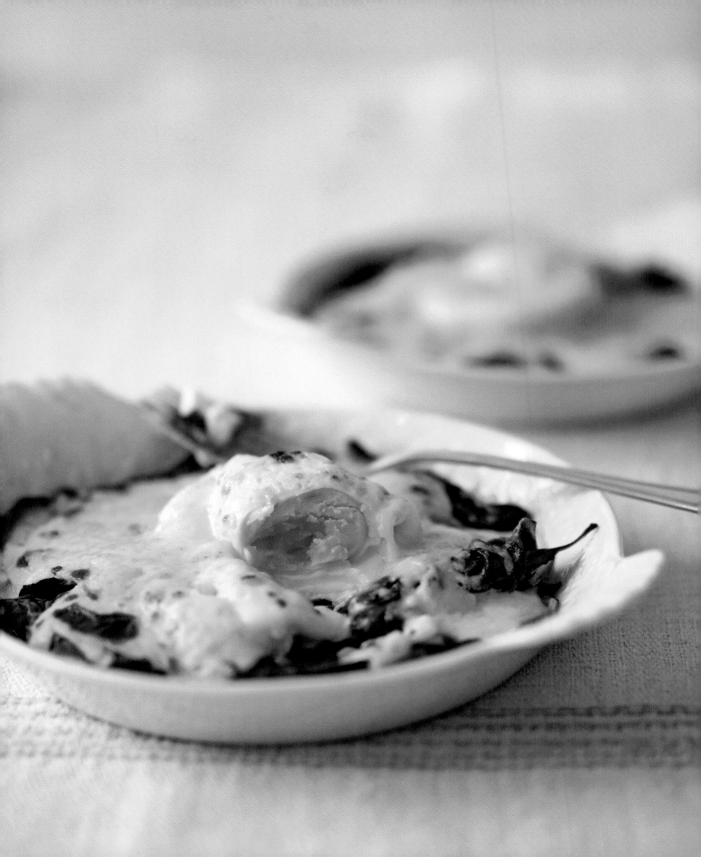

1 tablespoon butter

3 large eggs

1 tablespoon lactose-free or plant-based milk (limit soy to ¼ cup per portion), or standard milk if you know you tolerate lactose

1 tablespoon cream (optional)

1 to 1½oz smoked salmon, cut into narrow strips

1 teaspoon finely snipped chives

1 to 2 slices of toasted gluten-free bread

salt and freshly ground black pepper

SMOKED SALMON SCRAMBLED EGGS

PREPARATION TIME: 5 MINUTES
COOKING TIME: 3 TO 4 MINUTES
SERVES: 1

Melt the butter in a saucepan over very low heat until it is foaming.

Put the eggs into a bowl and beat well with a fork. Add the milk and season with salt and pepper.

Pour the egg mixture into the foaming butter and cook, stirring constantly with a wooden spoon, scraping the bottom of the pan and bringing the egg from the outside to the center. The eggs are done when they form soft, creamy curds and are barely set.

Remove the pan from the heat and stir in the cream, if using, the salmon, and the chives. Pile the mixture onto the hot toast on a warmed serving plate. Serve immediately.

2 cups peeled, chopped potatoes

2 tablespoons unsalted butter

1/3 cup rice flour, plus extra for dusting

pinch of salt

1 teaspoon gluten-free baking powder

1 egg, beaten

2 tablespoons olive oil

TO SERVE

butter

10½oz smoked salmon

snipped chives

POTATO SCONES WITH SMOKED SALMON

PREPARATION TIME: 10 MINUTES
COOKING TIME: 25 MINUTES
SERVES: 4

Cook the potatoes in a saucepan of boiling water for 10 to 12 minutes, until tender. Drain the potatoes and transfer to a bowl. Add the butter and mash everything together until light and fluffy.

Sift in the flour, salt, and baking powder, then add the egg and mix into a dough. Turn out the dough onto a lightly floured work surface and roll it out to a thickness of about ¼ inch. Cut the dough into 8 wedges and prick them all over with a fork.

Heat the oil in a large skillet over medium heat. Add the wedges and cook for 4 to 5 minutes on each side, until golden. Transfer the cooked wedges to serving plates.

To serve, spread each scone with a little butter, top with smoked salmon, and scatter with some snipped chives.

2 tablespoons garlic-infused olive oil

2 red bell peppers, seeded and diced

1 bunch of scallions (green parts only), sliced

¾ teaspoon dried oregano

14oz can diced tomatoes

4 eggs

2 tablespoons crumbled feta cheese

4 pieces toasted gluten-free pitta bread, to serve

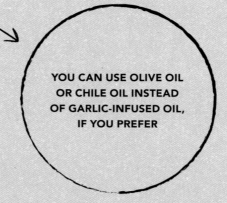

YOU CAN USE OLIVE OIL OR CHILE OIL INSTEAD OF GARLIC-INFUSED OIL, IF YOU PREFER

HUEVOS RANCHEROS

PREPARATION TIME: 5 MINUTES
COOKING TIME: 15 MINUTES
SERVES: 4

Preheat the broiler on the highest setting.

Heat the oil in a skillet over medium heat. Add the bell peppers and cook for 3 to 4 minutes, until softened. Add the scallions and oregano and cook for 1 minute. Add the tomatoes and cook for a further 5 minutes. Pour the tomato mixture into a shallow ovenproof dish. Use the back of a spoon to make 4 dips, evenly spaced, in the mixture.

Crack the eggs into the dips in the tomato mixture, then sprinkle with the feta. Cook under the hot broiler for 3 to 4 minutes, or until the eggs are cooked to your liking. Serve with toasted pitta bread.

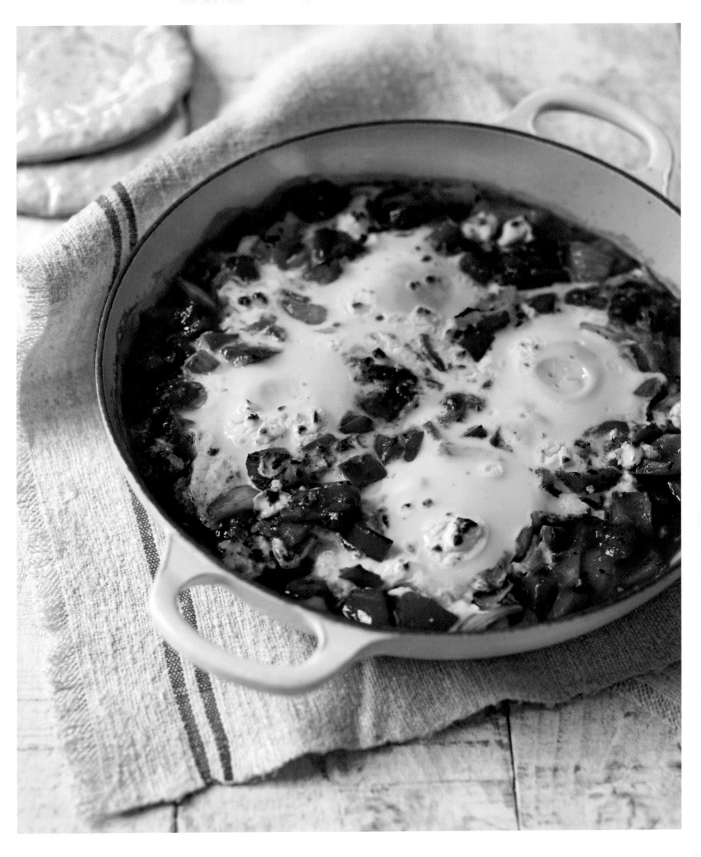

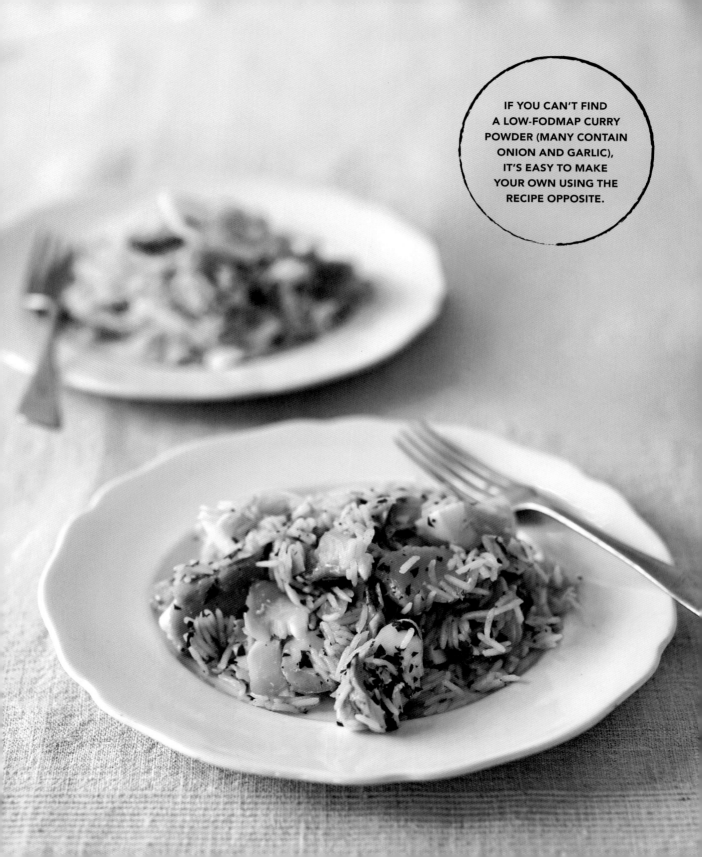

IF YOU CAN'T FIND A LOW-FODMAP CURRY POWDER (MANY CONTAIN ONION AND GARLIC), IT'S EASY TO MAKE YOUR OWN USING THE RECIPE OPPOSITE.

KEDGEREE

Place the haddock in a saucepan and cover with the measured water. Bring to a simmer, cover the pan with a lid, and cook over medium heat for 8 to 10 minutes. Drain the fish, reserving the cooking liquid, and keep the fish warm.

Heat the oil in the same saucepan you used to cook the fish, then add the scallions and cook for 1 to 2 minutes, until softened. Stir in the curry powder, then the rice.

Pour in 2 cups of the reserved cooking liquid and bring to a simmer, then cover the pan with a lid and cook for 15 minutes or until the rice is tender and the water has been absorbed.

Skin and flake the fish and carefully stir it into the rice with the quartered eggs.

Serve scattered with chopped parsley and sprinkled with a squeeze of lemon juice.

PREPARATION TIME: 10 MINUTES
COOKING TIME: 30 MINUTES
SERVES: 4

1lb 2oz smoked haddock

2½ cups water

3 tablespoons olive oil or canola oil

1 bunch of scallions (green parts only), sliced

¾ teaspoon mild Low-FODMAP Curry Powder (see below)

1 cup basmati rice

4 eggs, hard-cooked, peeled, and quartered

2 tablespoons chopped flat-leaf parsley

2 tablespoons lemon juice

LOW-FODMAP CURRY POWDER

Ensure that the curry powder you use is FODMAP friendly. Many products contain onion and garlic, which should be avoided in a low-FODMAP diet. If you can't find a low-FODMAP curry powder, you might like to make your own using the following recipe.

Combine 2 tablespoons each of ground cardamom, ground coriander, ground cumin, turmeric, and mustard powder with 1 teaspoon each of ground ginger and ground cinnamon, and ¼ to 2 teaspoons of cayenne pepper (depending on how hot you like your curries). Seal in an airtight container to store.

LUNCHES

CHICKEN CLUB SANDWICH ⟶

Heat the oil in a nonstick skillet over medium heat. Add the chicken and bacon and fry for 6 to 8 minutes, turning once or twice, until golden and cooked through.

Toast the bread, then spread 1 side of each piece with the mayonnaise. Divide the chicken and bacon across 4 slices of the toast, then top with the sliced cheese. Cover the cheese with 4 more slices of toast, then add the tomato slices and watercress. Complete the sandwich stacks with the final slices of toast.

Press the sandwiches together, then cut each stack into 4 small triangles. Secure with wooden toothpicks, if needed, and serve immediately.

PREPARATION TIME: 15 MINUTES
COOKING TIME: 10 MINUTES
SERVES: 4

1 tablespoon sunflower oil

4 small boneless, skinless chicken breasts, thinly sliced

8 slices smoked Canadian bacon

12 slices of gluten-free bread

1/4 cup mayonnaise (free from garlic and onion)

4 1/2 oz blue cheese, thinly sliced

4 vine tomatoes, thinly sliced

1 cup watercress

BLT SANDWICH

PREPARATION TIME: 5 MINUTES
COOKING TIME: 5 MINUTES
SERVES: 1

2 slices lean bacon

2 slices of gluten-free brown bread

2 tablespoons mayonnaise (free from garlic and onion)

2 vine tomatoes, halved

about 4 small romaine lettuce leaves

salt and freshly ground black pepper

Heat a small nonstick skillet and cook the bacon over medium heat for about 5 minutes, turning once, until it is golden brown and crisp. Remove and drain on paper towels.

Toast the bread. Spread 1 side of each piece of toast with mayonnaise and arrange the bacon, tomatoes, and lettuce on top. Season with salt and pepper and top with the remaining piece of toast. Cut the sandwich into quarters. Serve hot or cold.

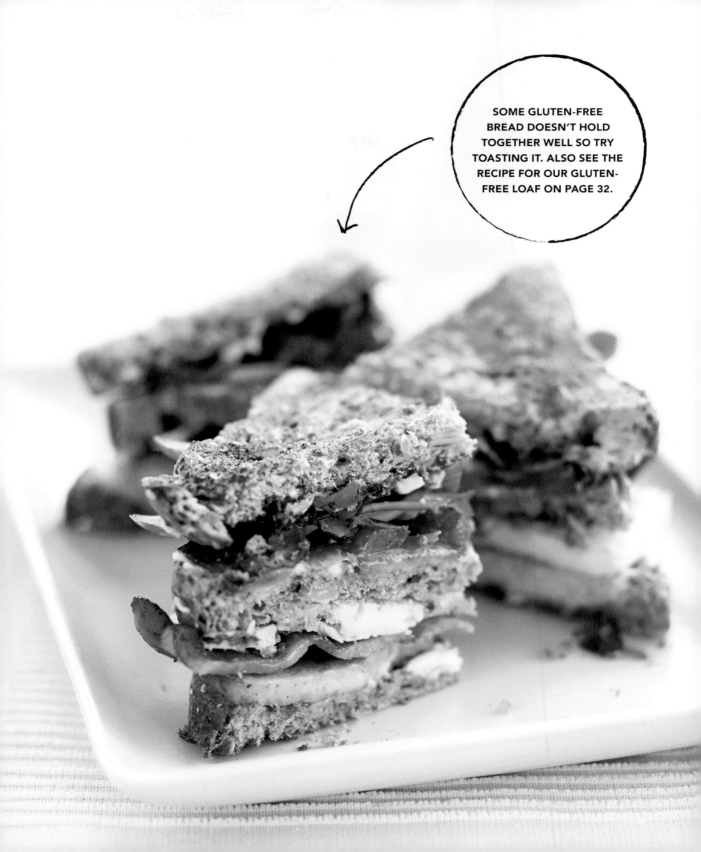

SOME GLUTEN-FREE BREAD DOESN'T HOLD TOGETHER WELL SO TRY TOASTING IT. ALSO SEE THE RECIPE FOR OUR GLUTEN-FREE LOAF ON PAGE 32.

1lb 2oz thick sirloin steak, trimmed

1 tablespoon olive oil

4 gluten-free mini baguettes or bread rolls, split open

4 sprigs of fresh cilantro

4 sprigs of basil or Thai basil

4 sprigs of mint

salt and freshly ground black pepper

FOR THE DRESSING

2 tablespoons Thai fish sauce

2 tablespoons lime juice

2 tablespoons soft light brown sugar

1 large red chile, thinly sliced

CHILE THAI BEEF BAGUETTES

PREPARATION TIME: 5 MINUTES, PLUS RESTING
COOKING TIME: 4 MINUTES
SERVES: 4

Heat a ridged grill pan until very hot.

Brush the steak with the oil and season liberally with salt and pepper. Add the steak to the hot pan and cook over high heat for 2 minutes on each side, ensuring you sear the steak all over. Let rest for 5 minutes, then cut it into thin slices. The steak should be rare.

Meanwhile, make the dressing. Put the fish sauce, lime juice, and sugar into a bowl and stir in the chile until the sugar has dissolved.

Fill the split rolls with the herbs and the beef slices along with any juices. Carefully drizzle the steak with the dressing and serve.

7oz rice noodles

1 bunch of scallions
(green parts only),
thinly sliced

¾-inch piece of fresh ginger
root, peeled and grated

1 red chile, finely chopped

2 tablespoons chopped fresh
cilantro

1 tablespoon chopped mint

¼ cucumber, cut into fine
matchsticks

2 x 6oz cans crabmeat,
drained, or 10½oz
fresh white crabmeat

1 tablespoon sesame oil

1 teaspoon Thai fish sauce

16 rice paper wrappers

THE WHITE BULBS OF SCALLIONS ARE HIGH IN FODMAPS SO BE SURE TO USE THE GREEN PARTS ONLY.

CRAB & NOODLE ASIAN WRAPS

**PREPARATION TIME: 15 MINUTES,
    PLUS STANDING**
COOKING TIME: 5 MINUTES
SERVES: 4

Cook the rice noodles following the package directions. Drain the noodles, then refresh under cold running water.

Mix together the remaining ingredients, except the rice paper wrappers, in a large bowl. Add the noodles and toss to mix. Cover and set aside for 10 minutes to allow the flavors to develop, then transfer to a serving dish.

Serve the filling mixture in a bowl alongside the rice paper wrappers and a bowl of warm water. Allow 4 rice paper wrappers per person and invite diners to soak and then top each wrapper with some of the crab and noodle mixture, roll it up, and enjoy.

PREPARATION TIME: 15 MINUTES,
    PLUS COOLING
COOKING TIME: ABOUT
    15 MINUTES
SERVES: 4

$1\frac{1}{2}$ cups sushi rice
....
2 tablespoons rice wine vinegar
....
1 tablespoon superfine sugar
....
2 sheets of nori
....
1 teaspoon wasabi
....
2 long strips of cucumber, cut to the length of the nori sheet and about $\frac{1}{2}$ inch in thickness
....
$3\frac{1}{2}$oz smoked salmon
....
2 tablespoons Japanese pickled ginger
....
$\frac{1}{4}$ cup light soy sauce

SALMON & CUCUMBER SUSHI

Cook the sushi rice following the package directions.

Mix together the vinegar and sugar in a bowl and stir until the sugar dissolves.

Once the rice is cooked, while it is still warm, mix in enough of the vinegar-and-sugar mixture to coat the rice grains, but do not allow the rice to become wet. Spread the rice out on a tray to cool quickly.

Take 1 nori sheet and place it on a bamboo mat with the longest edge parallel to the work surface and the ridged surface facing upward. With damp hands, cover three-quarters of the nori sheet with a thin layer of rice, leaving a band of nori at the edge farthest from you free of rice. Spread half of the wasabi in a line across the front edge of the rice. Place the cucumber strips and half the smoked salmon over the wasabi. Using the bamboo mat, roll up the nori, tucking in the cucumber and salmon as you go. Once you have rolled up the majority of the nori, wet your finger and dampen the clear edge of the nori sheet, then finish rolling up the nori. The wet edge will stick the roll together. Repeat with the remaining nori sheet, wasabi, cucumber, and salmon.

Using a sharp knife, cut the rolls into 8 even pieces.

Serve the pickled ginger and soy sauce alongside the nori rolls.

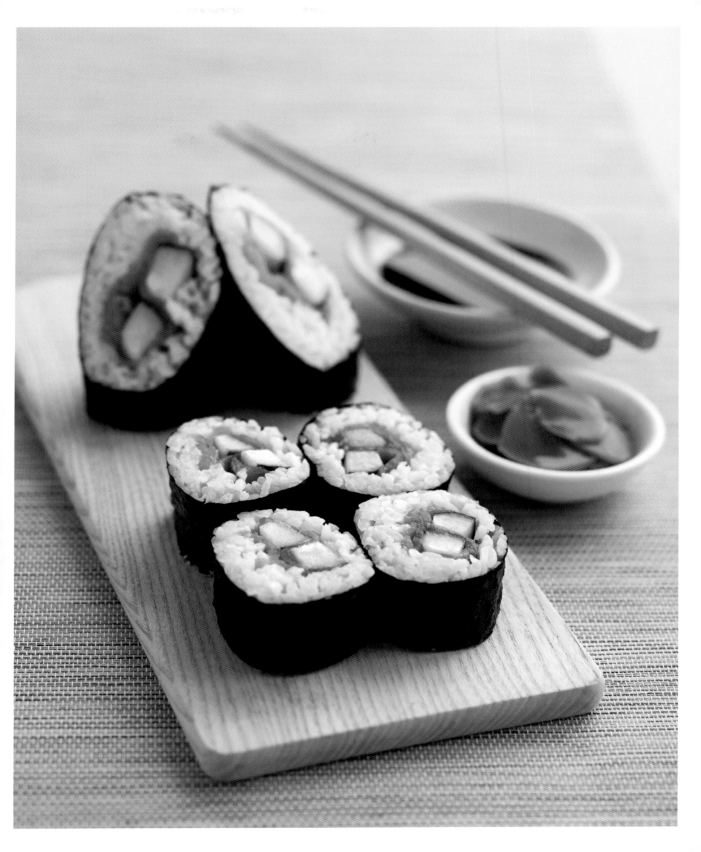

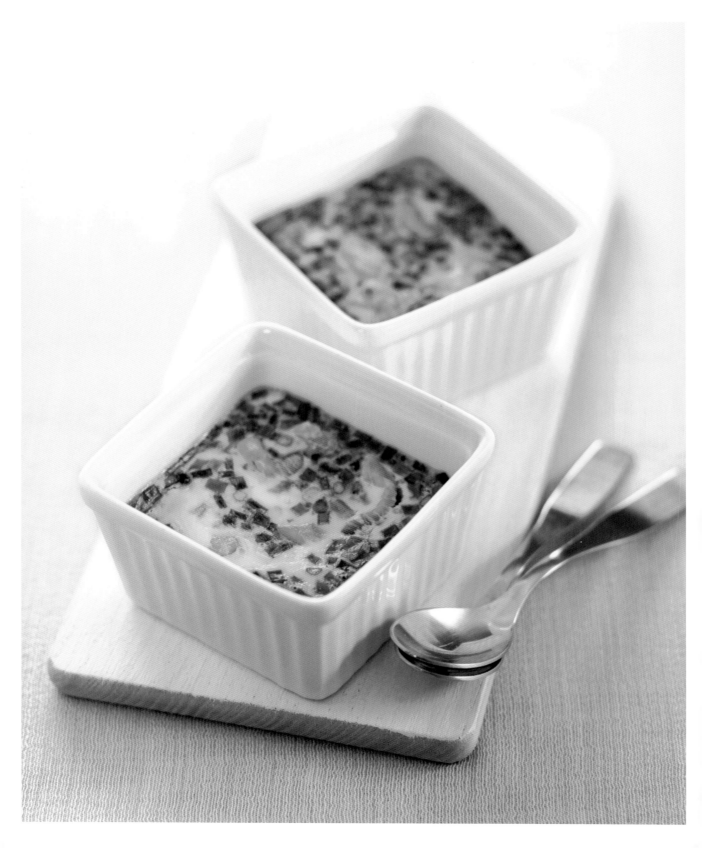

1 teaspoon unsalted butter

4¹⁄₂oz smoked salmon or
smoked trout, cut into
bite-sized pieces

2 large eggs

2 tablespoons cream

1 tablespoon chopped herbs
(such as chervil and chives)

salt and freshly ground
black pepper

toasted gluten-free bread,
to serve (optional)

IT IS A WIDELY
HELD MISCONCEPTION
THAT CREAM CONTAINS
A HIGH LACTOSE LOAD. IT IS,
IN FACT, NATURALLY
RELATIVELY LOW IN LACTOSE
SO IS SUITABLE FOR A
LOW-FODMAP DIET.

BAKED EGGS WITH SALMON

PREPARATION TIME: 5 MINUTES
COOKING TIME: 10 MINUTES
SERVES: 2

Preheat the oven to 400°F. Grease 2 ramekins, each with a capacity of 5fl oz, with the butter. Divide the salmon between the ramekins, then break in the eggs.

Mix together the cream and herbs in a bowl and season to taste with salt and pepper. Pour the seasoned cream into the ramekins and place them in a baking pan.

Half-fill the pan with boiling water, ensuring the water does not reach the rims of the ramekins, and transfer the pan to the oven. Bake for about 10 minutes, until the mixture is just set. Serve with triangles of crunchy fresh toast, if liked.

8 large eggs

1 teaspoon dried oregano

1 tablespoon finely chopped mint

1/4 cup finely chopped flat-leaf parsley

1 handful of fresh chives, snipped

2 tablespoons olive oil

2 large ripe vine tomatoes, coarsely chopped

1/2 zucchini, coarsely chopped

3/4 cup black olives, pitted

2/3 cup crumbled feta cheese

salt and freshly ground black pepper

crisp green salad, to serve (optional)

GREEK-STYLE SUMMER OMELET

PREPARATION TIME: 15 MINUTES
COOKING TIME: 15 MINUTES
SERVES: 4

Beat the eggs in a bowl and add the oregano, mint, parsley, and chives. Season well.

Heat the oil in a large, nonstick ovenproof skillet. Add the tomatoes, zucchini, and olives and cook for 3 to 4 minutes or until the vegetables begin to soften.

Meanwhile, preheat the broiler on a medium-high setting.

Reduce the heat under the skillet to medium and pour the eggs into the skillet. Cook for 3 to 4 minutes, stirring as they begin to set, until they are firm but still slightly runny in places.

Scatter the eggs with the feta, then place the skillet under the broiler and cook for 4 to 5 minutes or until the omelet is puffed up and golden. Cut it into wedges and serve with a crisp green salad, if liked.

**PREPARATION TIME: 30 MINUTES,
    PLUS CHILLING AND COOLING
COOKING TIME: 30 TO 35 MINUTES
MAKES: 6**

1 cup rice flour, plus
extra for dusting

pinch of salt

1 stick butter, plus
extra for greasing

2 egg yolks

2 teaspoons cold water

FOR THE FILLING

1 tablespoon sunflower oil

4 slices smoked bacon, about
2¾oz in total, diced

1 cup grated sharp
Cheddar cheese, divided

3 eggs

1 cup lactose-free or plant-
based milk (limit soy to
¼ cup per portion), or
standard milk if you know
you tolerate lactose

2 teaspoons mustard powder

2 tablespoons snipped
chives (optional)

salt and freshly ground
black pepper

salad, to serve

THIS DISH MAKES A
FANTASTIC LOW-FODMAP
CARRY-TO-WORK LUNCH, AS
IT IS EASILY TRANSPORTABLE
AND CAN BE ENJOYED
HOT OR COLD.

QUICHES LORRAINE

Preheat the oven to 375°F. Grease 6 individual 4-inch loose-bottomed fluted tart pans.

For the pastry, put the rice flour, salt, and butter into a bowl and rub in with your fingertips until you have fine crumbs. Add the egg yolks and mix to a soft dough, adding the water as required.

Cut the pastry into 6 equal portions, then roll out 1 portion between 2 sheets of plastic wrap until it is a little larger than one of the prepared tart pans. Remove the top sheet of plastic wrap, turn the pastry over, drape it into the pan, and remove the other sheet of plastic wrap. Press the pastry into the bottom and sides of the pan with fingers dusted in rice flour. Trim off the excess pastry a little above the rim of the pan. Repeat with the remaining pastry

portions until 6 tart shells have been made. Place these on a cookie sheet and chill for 15 minutes.

Meanwhile, make the filling. Heat the oil in a skillet over medium-high heat. Add the bacon and fry for 5 minutes, stirring, until golden.

Divide three-quarters of the cheese between the tart shells, then scatter the bacon on top.

Beat the eggs, milk, and mustard in a large measuring cup with a little salt and pepper, then pour the mixture into the tart shells. Scatter with the chives, if using, and the remaining cheese. Bake for 25 to 30 minutes, until the tops are golden and the pastry shells are cooked through. Let cool for 5 minutes, then remove from the pans and serve with salad.

3¾ cups boiling water

2 to 3 dried red chiles

2 teaspoons cumin seeds

1 teaspoon coriander seeds

1 teaspoon saffron threads

small bunch of flat-leaf parsley (use leaves and stems), plus extra leaves, torn, to garnish

small bunch of fresh cilantro (use leaves and stems), plus extra leaves, torn, to garnish

small bunch of mint

4 to 6 peppercorns

1 teaspoon sea salt

whole chiles, to garnish (optional)

ALTHOUGH CHILES ARE LOW IN FODMAPS, SOME PEOPLE FIND THEY MAKE THEIR DIGESTIVE SYMPTOMS FLARE UP. OMIT THE CHILE IN THIS RECIPE IF YOU KNOW IT DOESN'T SUIT YOU.

SIMPLE HERB, CHILE & SAFFRON BROTH

PREPARATION TIME: 5 MINUTES
COOKING TIME: 10 MINUTES
SERVES: 4

Pour the measured water into a saucepan set over medium heat. Add the remaining ingredients and boil gently for 8 to 10 minutes.

Strain and discard the herbs. Serve the broth between courses or as a digestive, garnished with herbs and whole chiles, if liked.

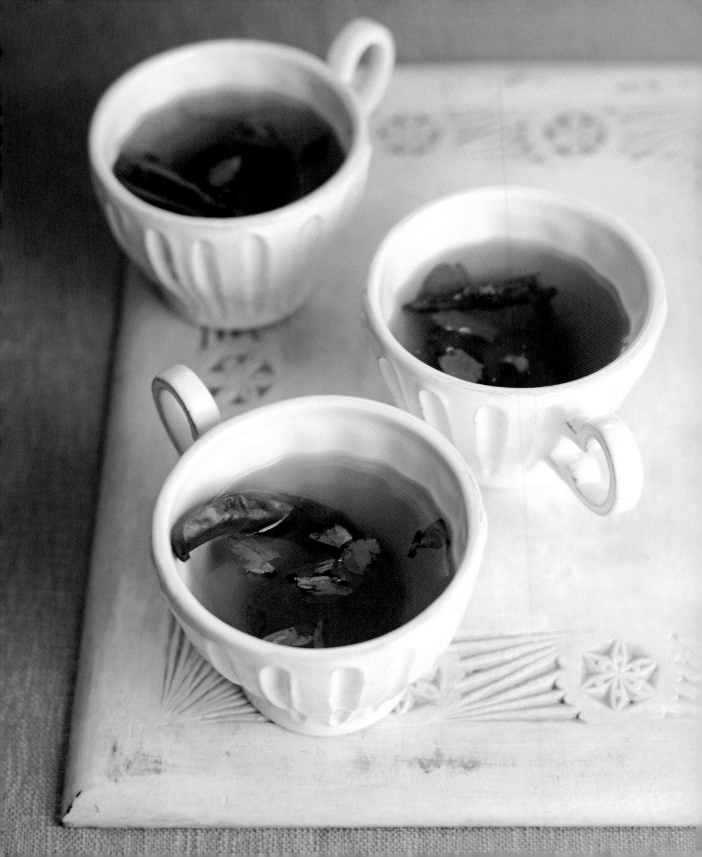

QUICK CHICKEN SOUP

Put the chicken wings, tomatoes, potatoes, scallions, herbs, and spices into a large Dutch oven. Pour in the stock or measured water, add salt to taste, and bring to a boil. Cook over medium heat for 25 minutes.

Remove and discard the herbs. Remove and reserve the chicken wings. Strain the vegetables, reserving the stock, and pass them through a food mill or process in a blender until smooth.

Return the blended vegetables, the stock, and the chicken wings to the casserole and bring to a boil. Add the rice in a steady stream, stir, and cook over medium heat for a further 5 minutes. Serve immediately.

PREPARATION TIME: 10 MINUTES
COOKING TIME: 30 MINUTES
SERVES: 6

8 chicken wings

3 vine tomatoes

2 potatoes, peeled and halved

1 bunch of scallions (green parts only), sliced

1 tied bunch of flat-leaf parsley

1 tied bunch of fresh cilantro

¼ teaspoon freshly ground black pepper

¼ teaspoon ground turmeric

5 quarts low-FODMAP chicken or vegetable stock (see below) or water

¼ cup short-grain rice

salt

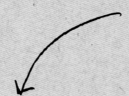

LOW-FODMAP VEGETABLE STOCK

Many stocks contain onion and garlic, which should be avoided in a low-FODMAP diet. If you can't find a low-FODMAP version, you might like to make your own using the following recipe.

Heat 2 tablespoons of garlic-infused olive oil in a large saucepan or stockpot. Add 4 large carrots and 2 celery stalks, chopped, and cover with a lid. Let sweat over medium heat for about 10 minutes, until soft. Add 3 quarts water, followed by 3 bay leaves, 3 to 4 sprigs of mixed herbs (such as rosemary, thyme, lemon thyme, and parsley), a small bunch of chives, 10 peppercorns, and a large pinch of salt. Bring to a boil, then gently simmer for 2 hours. Strain the stock. Either use it immediately or let cool, then freeze the stock in ice-cube trays and store in the freezer for up to 3 months for readily available low-FODMAP stock.

2¼lb lean beef for stew, diced

½lb boneless lean pork, diced

2½ quarts water

24 okra, trimmed and chopped (limit each portion to 2¼oz)

1lb 2oz kale, tough stalks discarded, coarsely chopped

2 green bell peppers, seeded and chopped

sprig of thyme

¼ teaspoon cayenne pepper

2 small sweet potatoes, peeled and diced (limit each portion to 2½oz)

2¾ cups peeled, sliced potatoes

2 scallions (green parts only), coarsely chopped

salt

gluten-free crusty bread, to serve (optional)

LIMIT OKRA TO 6 PODS PER SERVING TO ENSURE THIS DISH REMAINS LOW-FODMAP-DIET FRIENDLY.

JAMAICAN PEPPER POT SOUP

PREPARATION TIME: 20 MINUTES
COOKING TIME: 1 HOUR 10 MINUTES
SERVES: 6

Put the meat and measured water into a large saucepan. Bring to a boil, then reduce the heat, partially cover the pan with a lid, and let simmer for about 30 minutes.

Add the okra, kale, and green bell peppers to the saucepan with the thyme and cayenne pepper. Partially cover the pan again and simmer over medium heat for 15 minutes.

Tip in the sweet potatoes, potato slices, and scallions and let simmer for a further 20 minutes or until the potatoes are tender and the meat is cooked through. Add more water if the soup is too thick. Season with salt and serve in warmed soup bowls with gluten-free crusty bread, if liked.

¾ cup gluten-free
all-purpose flour

2 teaspoons ground cumin

1 teaspoon chile powder

2 teaspoons dried oregano

1 cup cold water

14oz white fish, skinned and
sliced into thick strips

vegetable oil, for deep-frying

salt and freshly ground
black pepper

FOR THE TARTARE SAUCE

½ cup mayonnaise
(free from garlic and onion)

1 fresh jalapeño pepper,
seeded, if liked, and diced

1 teaspoon capers, drained

1 small gherkin (free from
celery seeds), finely chopped

grated zest and juice of
½ lime

handful of fresh cilantro
leaves, chopped

TO SERVE

¼ red cabbage

8 gluten-free corn tortillas
(free from pea protein)

FISH TACOS WITH TARTARE SAUCE

PREPARATION TIME: 20 MINUTES
COOKING TIME: 10 TO 15 MINUTES
SERVES: 4

Place the flour, spices, oregano, and measured water in a shallow dish and stir together until the mixture resembles heavy cream. Season the fish, then dip it in the flour mixture and shake the dish until the fish pieces are well coated.

Fill a large saucepan with the oil to a depth of one-third. Heat to 350 to 375°F or until a cube of bread immersed in the oil browns in 15 seconds. Allow any excess coating to drop off of the fish, then deep-fry the fish in batches for 3 to 5 minutes, until golden and crisp. Remove from the pan, drain on paper towels, and keep warm.

To make the tartare sauce, mix the mayonnaise, chile, capers, and gherkin in a bowl. Add the lime zest and juice to taste, reserving a dash of lime juice with which to dress the cabbage, then stir in the cilantro.

Toss the cabbage with a little salt and the reserved lime juice. Divide the cabbage among the tortillas, then add the deep-fried fish. Drizzle with the tartare sauce and serve immediately.

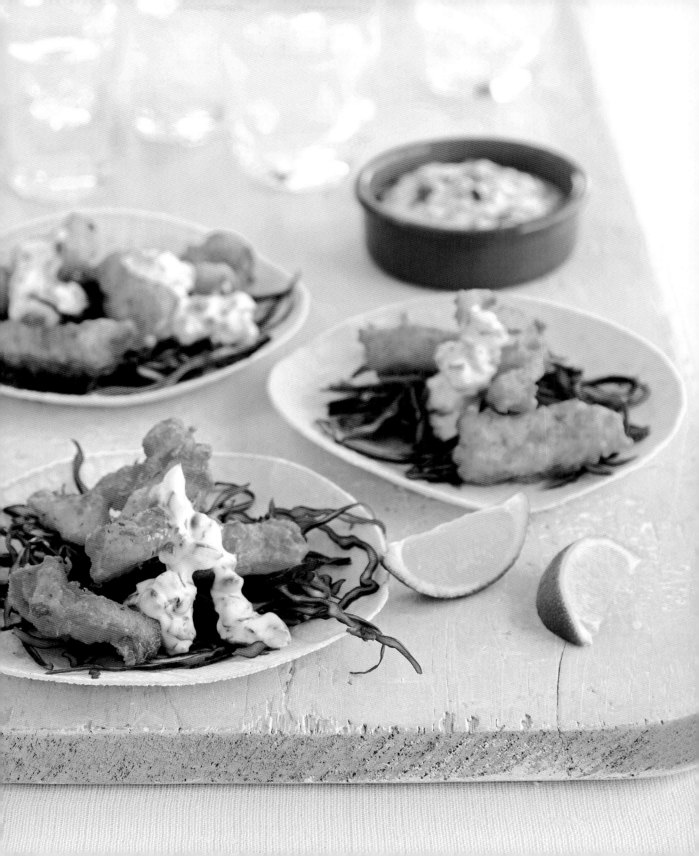

2 skinless chicken breasts, halved horizontally

2 tablespoons gluten-free all-purpose flour

1 egg, beaten

1¼ cups gluten-free bread crumbs

¾ cup freshly grated Parmesan cheese

3 tablespoons sunflower oil

4 small gluten-free bread rolls, split open

¼ cup mayonnaise (free from garlic and onion)

4 small handfuls of green salad leaves

salt and freshly ground black pepper

CHECK THAT YOUR MAYONNAISE CONTAINS NO HIDDEN ONION OR GARLIC UNDER THE GUISE OF "FLAVORINGS." IF THE LABEL DOES NOT SPECIFY WHICH FLAVORINGS ARE USED, AVOID USING THE PRODUCT.

PARMESAN CHICKEN SCALLOPS

PREPARATION TIME: 20 MINUTES
COOKING TIME: 5 MINUTES
SERVES: 4

Place the chicken halves between 2 pieces of plastic wrap and beat with a rolling pin to flatten slightly.

Put the flour onto a plate and the beaten egg into a shallow dish. On a separate plate, mix together the bread crumbs and grated Parmesan and season with salt and pepper.

Lightly coat each piece of chicken in flour, then shake off any excess flour and dip each piece into the beaten egg. Next, roll it in the bread-crumb mixture to coat, pressing the bread crumbs on firmly.

Heat the oil in a large skillet over medium heat. Add the chicken and cook for about 5 minutes, turning once, until golden, crisp, and cooked through.

Spread the bread rolls with mayonnaise, then fill with salad leaves and the hot chicken. Serve immediately.

PREPARATION TIME: 25 MINUTES, PLUS COOLING

COOKING TIME: 35 MINUTES

MAKES: 4

1 tablespoon garlic-infused olive oil, plus extra for greasing

1 zucchini, diced

1 bunch of scallions (green parts only), chopped

½ yellow bell pepper, seeded and diced

½ red bell pepper, seeded and diced

14oz can diced tomatoes

1 tablespoon chopped rosemary or basil

½ teaspoon superfine sugar

beaten egg, to glaze

salt and freshly ground black pepper

salad, to serve

FOR THE PASTRY

1½ cups gluten-free bread flour

¾ stick butter, diced

½ cup diced sharp Cheddar cheese, plus extra, grated, for sprinkling

2 egg yolks

salt and freshly ground black pepper

PICNIC PIES WITH CHEESE

To make the pie filling, heat the oil in a saucepan, add the zucchini, scallions, and diced bell peppers and fry briefly, then add the tomatoes, herbs, sugar, and a little salt and pepper. Simmer, uncovered, for 10 minutes, stirring from time to time, until thickened. Let cool.

Preheat the oven to 375°F. Grease a large cookie sheet.

To make the pastry, put the flour, butter, and a little salt and pepper into a bowl and rub in the butter until the mixture resembles fine bread crumbs. Stir in the cheese. Add the egg yolks and 2 teaspoons water and mix to form a smooth dough.

Knead the dough lightly, then cut it into 4 pieces. Roll out 1 of the pieces between 2 sheets of plastic wrap and pat it into a neat 7-inch circle. Remove the top sheet of plastic wrap and spoon one-quarter of the filling into the center of the circle. Brush the

pastry edges with beaten egg, then fold the pastry circle in half, using the lower sheet of plastic wrap to help you if necessary. Peel the pastry off the plastic wrap, lift it onto the prepared cookie sheet, then press the edges together well to seal the pie. Press together any breaks in the pastry. Repeat with the remaining pastry pieces and filling until 4 pies have been made.

Brush the prepared pies with beaten egg, sprinkle with a little extra cheese, then bake for 20 minutes, until golden brown. Transfer the pies to a wire rack. Serve warm or cold with salad.

oil, for greasing

1lb 2oz good-quality pork sausagemeat

2 teaspoons ground cumin

2 teaspoons ground coriander

2 teaspoons fennel seeds

1 tablespoon ground paprika

1 tablespoon garlic-infused oil

2 scallions (green parts only), finely chopped

gluten-free flour, for dusting

1lb 2oz ready-made gluten-free puff pastry

beaten egg, to glaze

salt and freshly ground black pepper

MERGUEZ SAUSAGE ROLLS

PREPARATION TIME: 25 MINUTES
COOKING TIME: 25 TO 30 MINUTES
MAKES: 32

Preheat the oven to 425°F. Grease a large cookie sheet with oil.

Put the sausagemeat into a bowl and add the cumin, coriander, fennel seeds, paprika, garlic-infused oil, scallions, and a little salt and pepper. Mix well with your hands until evenly combined.

Lightly dust your work surface with flour, then roll out the pastry thinly on the floured surface to a 16-inch square. Cut the square into 4 strips. Divide the pork mixture into 4 portions and pinch out a portion of the meat mixture along the center of each strip. Brush the pastry edges with a little beaten egg and fold the pastry strip over the sausagemeat to bring the long edges together. Press the edges of the pastry firmly together to make long, thin logs.

Brush the logs with beaten egg, then cut each log into 8 pieces, each about 2 inches long. Transfer the pieces to the prepared cookie sheet. Score 2 or 3 cuts along the top of each piece using a sharp knife. Bake for 15 minutes, then reduce the oven temperature to 325°F and bake for a further 10 to 15 minutes, until deep golden and cooked through.

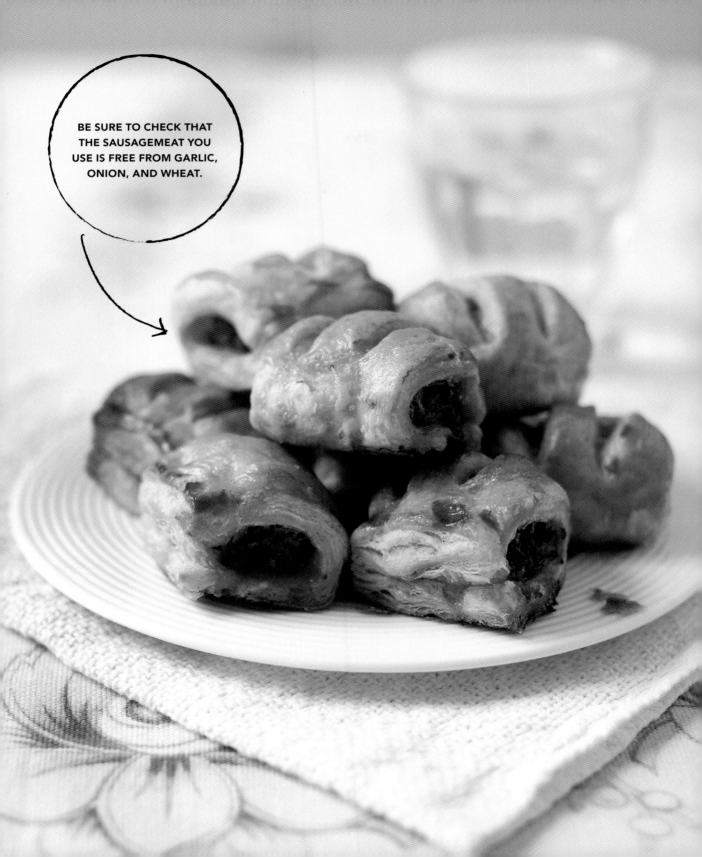

BE SURE TO CHECK THAT THE SAUSAGEMEAT YOU USE IS FREE FROM GARLIC, ONION, AND WHEAT.

1½ cups gluten-free all-purpose flour

2 teaspoons gluten-free baking powder

½ cup polenta or cornmeal

2 tablespoons chopped flat-leaf parsley

1 cup finely grated sharp Cheddar cheese, divided

2 tablespoons capers, drained and rinsed

1 teaspoon salt

1 teaspoon freshly ground black pepper

1 large egg

¾ stick butter, melted

1 cup lactose-free or plant-based milk (limit soy to ¼ cup per portion), or standard milk if you know you tolerate lactose

CAPER, CHEESE & POLENTA MUFFINS

PREPARATION TIME: 15 MINUTES, PLUS COOLING
COOKING TIME: 20 TO 25 MINUTES
MAKES: 10

Preheat the oven to 375°F. Line a 12-hole muffin pan with 10 paper muffin cups.

Sift the flour and baking powder together into a large bowl. Add the polenta or cornmeal, parsley, three-quarters of the cheese, the capers, salt, and pepper and mix well.

Beat the egg, melted butter, and milk together in a separate bowl. Pour this mixture over the dry ingredients and stir until only just combined—the batter should be lumpy.

Spoon the mixture into the prepared muffin cups until about three-quarters full, then sprinkle the tops with the remaining grated cheese. Bake for 20 to 25 minutes, until risen and firm.

Let cool in the pan for 5 minutes, then transfer to a wire rack to cool further. Serve warm.

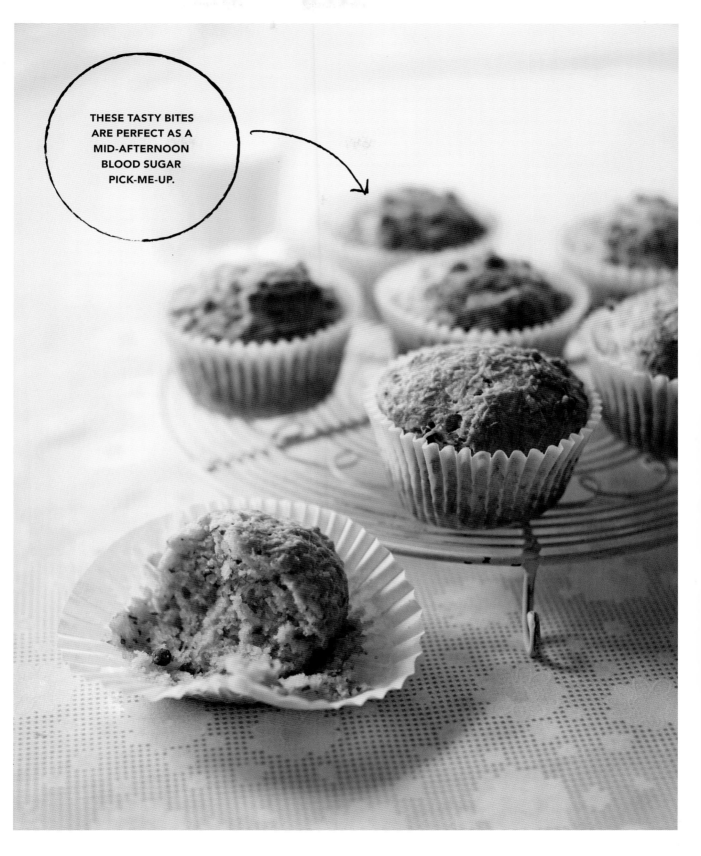

THESE TASTY BITES
ARE PERFECT AS A
MID-AFTERNOON
BLOOD SUGAR
PICK-ME-UP.

2 cups rolled oats

3 sprigs of rosemary, leaves stripped

1 cup gluten-free all-purpose flour, plus extra for dusting

1 teaspoon gluten-free baking powder

pinch of salt

¾ stick unsalted butter, cubed

½ cup lactose-free or plant-based milk (limit soy to ¼ cup per portion), or standard milk if you know you tolerate lactose

lactose-free cheese, to serve

TOP THESE WITH 1 TABLESPOON OF PEANUT OR ALMOND BUTTER, CHEESE, COLD MEATS, OR SMOKED SALMON AND CUCUMBER FOR A DELICIOUS SNACK.

HERBED OATCAKES

PREPARATION TIME: 10 MINUTES
COOKING TIME: 15 MINUTES
SERVES: 4

Preheat the oven to 375°F.

Put the oats and the rosemary leaves into the bowl of a food processor and process until they start to break down and the mixture resembles bread crumbs.

Add the flour, baking powder, and salt and blitz again. Add the butter and process until it is mixed in. Then, with the motor running, pour in the milk and process until the dough comes together in a ball.

Turn out the dough onto a lightly floured work surface and roll it out to a thickness of about ¼ inch. Cut out 20 to 24 disks using a cutter 1½ to 2 inches in diameter, rerolling the dough as necessary.

Arrange the dough disks on a cookie sheet. Bake for 12 to 15 minutes, until just starting to turn golden at the edges. Cool on a wire rack. Serve with cheese. Store in an airtight container for up to 7 days.

3¾ cups gluten-free strong white bread flour, plus extra for dusting
....
¼ cup polenta
....
2½ teaspoons fast-acting dry yeast
....
1 teaspoon salt
....
1½ cups warm water
....
⅓ cup olive oil, plus extra for greasing and brushing
....
1 teaspoon cumin seeds, plus extra to serve
....
1 red chile, seeded, if liked, and chopped, plus extra to serve
....
sea salt flakes, to serve (optional)

SPICY GRIDDLED FLATBREADS

PREPARATION TIME: 20 MINUTES, PLUS PROVING

COOKING TIME: 15 MINUTES

MAKES: 8

Place the flour, polenta, yeast, and salt in a bowl and mix together. Add the measured water, 3 tablespoons of the oil, the cumin seeds, and the chile. Mix together to form a dough. Knead the dough using an electric hand mixer for 5 minutes, or by hand on a lightly floured surface for 10 minutes, until the dough is soft and springy. Put the dough into a lightly oiled bowl, cover with plastic wrap, and let rise in a warm place for about 1 hour, or until the mixture has doubled in size.

Tip the dough out onto a lightly floured surface, then punch it down and knead a couple of times until the air is knocked out. Divide the mixture into 8 equal balls and keep loosely covered with lightly oiled plastic wrap. Roll out each ball until ¼ inch thick.

Heat a griddle until smoking hot. Brush the flatbreads with a little oil, then cook, in batches, for 3 to 5 minutes on each side, until lightly charred and cooked through. Tear the griddled flatbreads into large chunks and serve warm, scattered with a little chopped red chile, some cumin seeds, and sea salt flakes, if liked.

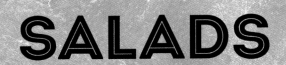

SALADS

½ head of white cabbage, thinly sliced

2 carrots, thinly sliced

¾ cup thinly sliced radishes

2 scallions (green parts only), thinly sliced

1 bunch of cilantro, chopped

FOR THE DRESSING

1 teaspoon cumin seeds

1 red chile, seeded, if liked, and finely chopped

grated zest and juice of 2 limes

2 tablespoons olive oil

salt and freshly ground black pepper

WHILE WHITE AND RED CABBAGE CAN BE ENJOYED ON A LOW-FODMAP DIET, SAVOY CABBAGE NEEDS TO BE LIMITED TO 1½OZ PER SITTING.

CRUNCHY VEGETABLE SALAD

PREPARATION TIME: 10 MINUTES, PLUS STANDING

SERVES: 4

To make the dressing, mix together all the ingredients in a bowl. Season well.

Put the salad ingredients into a serving bowl, add the dressing, and toss well. Let stand for 5 minutes before serving.

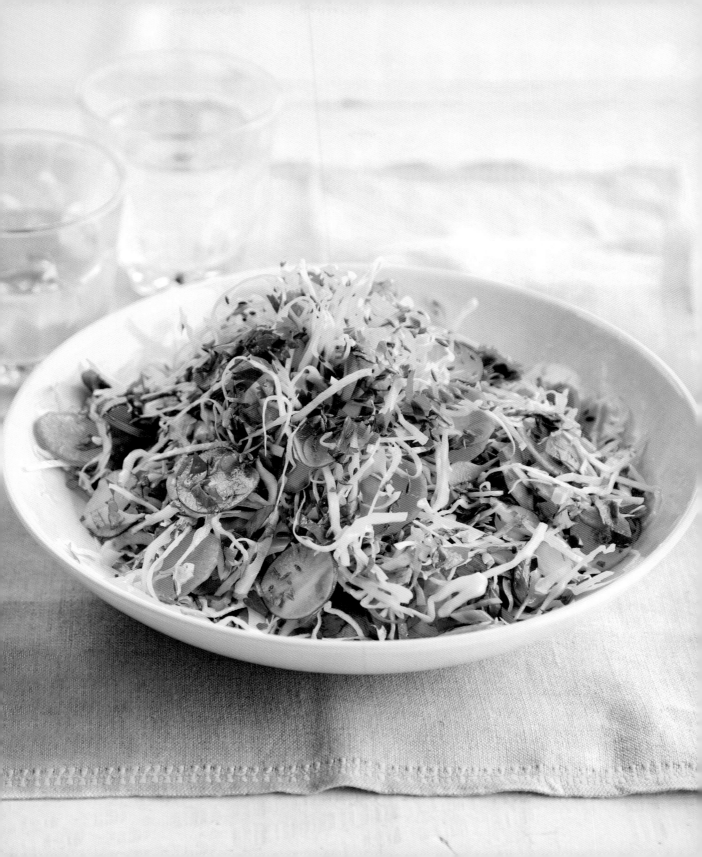

SALMON & WATERCRESS SALAD →

PREPARATION TIME: 10 MINUTES
SERVES: 4

Whisk together the oil, orange juice, mustard, and sugar in a small bowl to make a dressing.

In a large bowl, toss together the watercress, cucumber, orange segments, and walnuts. Add the smoked salmon and dressing and toss to coat well. Serve with toasted pitta bread, if liked.

3 tablespoons extra-virgin olive oil

juice of 1 orange

$\frac{1}{2}$ teaspoon mustard

$\frac{1}{2}$ teaspoon superfine sugar

$3\frac{1}{2}$oz watercress

$\frac{1}{2}$ cucumber, chopped

2 oranges, peeled and segmented

2 tablespoons toasted walnuts

6oz smoked salmon strips

4 pieces gluten-free pitta bread, toasted, to serve (optional)

SHRIMP & FENNEL SALAD
WITH BASIL CITRUS DRESSING

$\frac{1}{2}$ orange

$\frac{1}{2}$ lime

handful of snipped chives

$\frac{3}{4}$ cup loosely packed fresh basil leaves

$\frac{1}{4}$ cup extra-virgin olive oil

1 fennel bulb, thinly sliced (limit each portion to $1\frac{3}{4}$oz)

$3\frac{1}{2}$oz green salad leaves

$5\frac{1}{2}$oz cooked shelled jumbo shrimp

salt and freshly ground black pepper

PREPARATION TIME: 10 MINUTES
SERVES: 2

Squeeze the juice of the orange and lime into the bowl of a small food processor, add the chives and basil, and pulse briefly. With the motor running, slowly add the oil in a thin stream to make a smooth dressing, then season.

Arrange the remaining ingredients on serving plates. Drizzle each salad with the dressing and serve.

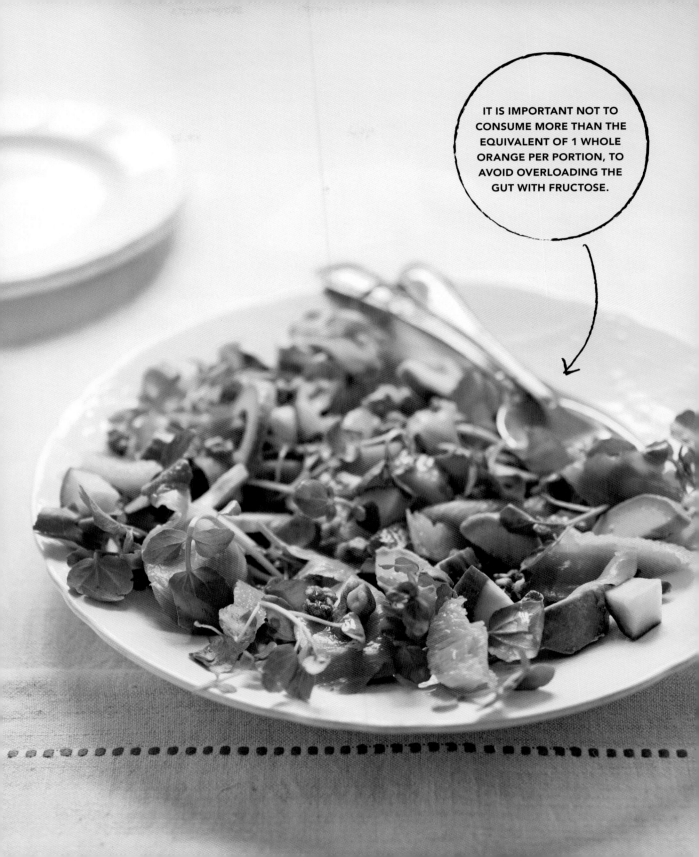

IT IS IMPORTANT NOT TO CONSUME MORE THAN THE EQUIVALENT OF 1 WHOLE ORANGE PER PORTION, TO AVOID OVERLOADING THE GUT WITH FRUCTOSE.

¾ cup quinoa

1 small yellow bell pepper, seeded and diced

1 small red bell pepper, seeded and diced

4 scallions (green parts only), sliced

⅓ cucumber, seeded and diced

½ fennel bulb, finely diced

2 tablespoons finely chopped curly parsley

2 tablespoons finely chopped mint

2 tablespoons finely chopped fresh cilantro

2 tablespoons sunflower seeds, divided

finely grated zest and juice of 2 limes

FOR THE DRESSING

4 teaspoons Low-FODMAP Harissa Paste (*see page 128*)

finely grated zest and juice of 2 limes

½ cup sunflower oil

salt and freshly ground black pepper

FENNEL IS LOW FODMAP ONLY IN SMALL AMOUNTS, SO ENSURE YOU LIMIT EACH PORTION TO 1¾OZ.

ZESTY QUINOA SALAD

PREPARATION TIME: 15 MINUTES
COOKING TIME: 15 TO 20 MINUTES
SERVES: 4

Put the quinoa into a saucepan of cold water, bring to a boil, and cook for 15 to 20 minutes or until the quinoa is translucent and just cooked. Drain and rinse thoroughly in cold water.

Meanwhile, make the dressing. Put the harissa paste, lime zest and juice, and oil into a bowl or large measuring cup and whisk well to blend. Season to taste and set aside.

Mix the quinoa in a large bowl with the prepared vegetables and herbs, 1 tablespoon of the sunflower seeds, and the lime juice and zest. Scatter with the remaining sunflower seeds and serve with the dressing.

MIDDLE-EASTERN BREAD SALAD

PREPARATION TIME: 10 MINUTES,
   PLUS COOLING
COOKING TIME: 2 TO 3 MINUTES
SERVES: 4 TO 6

2 gluten-free flatbreads or
gluten-free soft tortillas

1 large green bell pepper,
seeded and diced

1 small Lebanese cucumber
or ¼ regular cucumber, diced

½ lb cherry tomatoes, halved

1 handful of chives, finely
snipped

2 tablespoons chopped mint

2 tablespoons chopped flat-leaf
parsley

2 tablespoons chopped fresh
cilantro

3 tablespoons olive oil

¼ cup lemon juice

salt and freshly ground black
pepper

Toast the flatbreads or tortillas on a preheated griddle or under a preheated hot broiler for 2 to 3 minutes or until charred. Let cool, then tear into bite-sized pieces.

Put the green bell pepper, cucumber, tomatoes, and herbs into a serving bowl. Add the oil and lemon juice, season with salt and pepper, and toss well. Add the bread and stir again. Serve immediately.

7oz vermicelli rice noodles

½ cucumber, seeded and cut into matchsticks

1 carrot, cut into matchsticks

1¾ cups bean sprouts

4½oz green snap beans, cut into thin strips

2 tablespoons chopped fresh cilantro

2 tablespoons chopped mint

1 red chile, seeded and thinly sliced

2 tablespoons chopped blanched peanuts, to garnish

FOR THE DRESSING

1 tablespoon sunflower or peanut oil

½ teaspoon superfine sugar

1 tablespoon Thai fish sauce

2 tablespoons freshly squeezed lime juice

VIETNAMESE-STYLE VEGETABLE NOODLE SALAD

PREPARATION TIME: 20 MINUTES
COOKING TIME: 5 MINUTES
SERVES: 4

Bring a large saucepan of water to a boil, then turn off the heat and add the rice noodles. Cover and let cook for 4 minutes, until just tender (alternatively, cook them following the package directions). Drain the noodles and cool immediately in a bowl of ice-cold water.

To make the dressing, put the ingredients into a small bowl and stir until the sugar has dissolved.

Place the prepared vegetables, herbs, and chile in a large mixing bowl. Pour in half of the dressing and toss to combine.

Drain the noodles and transfer to four serving bowls. Heap the salad on top of the noodles and drizzle with the remaining dressing. Serve scattered with chopped peanuts.

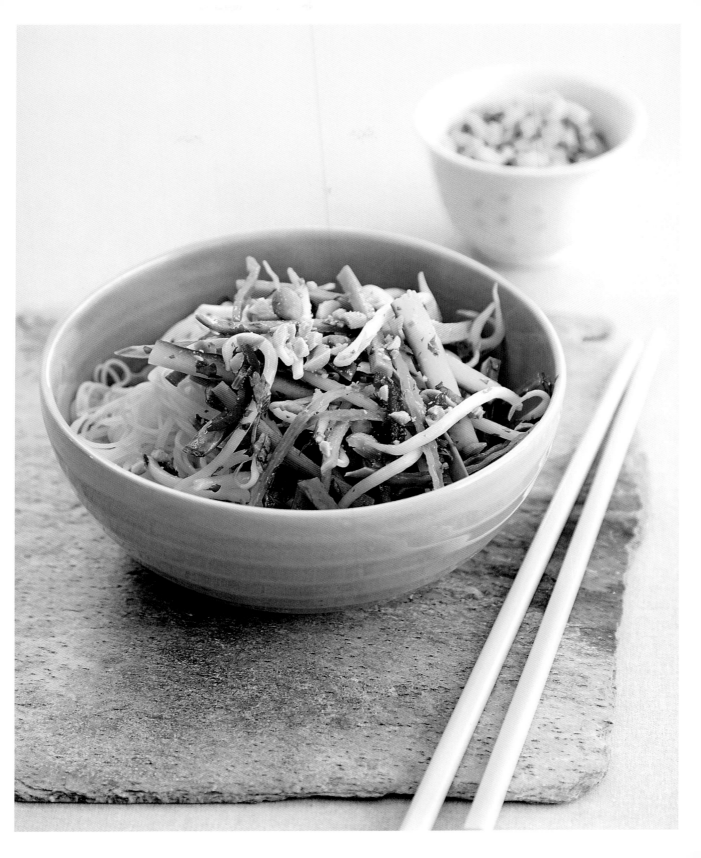

$1^2/_3$ cups halved cherry
tomatoes

1 tablespoon olive oil

$5^1/_2$oz mini mozzarella cheese
balls, drained

$2^1/_2$ tablespoons pine nuts,
toasted

sea salt and freshly ground
black pepper

gluten-free bread, to serve

FOR THE DRESSING

$^2/_3$ cup tightly packed arugula

12 basil leaves

$^1/_4$ cup extra-virgin olive oil,
divided

1 teaspoon red wine vinegar

sea salt and freshly ground
black pepper

ROAST TOMATO &
MOZZARELLA SALAD

**PREPARATION TIME: 10 MINUTES,
 PLUS COOLING
COOKING TIME: 20 MINUTES
SERVES: 4**

Preheat the oven to 400°F.

Place the tomatoes cut-side up in a small roasting pan. Drizzle with
the olive oil and season with a little sea salt and pepper. Roast for 20
minutes, until softened. Remove from the oven and let cool.

To make the dressing, put the arugula and basil leaves, 2 tablespoons
of the extra-virgin olive oil, and the vinegar into a small bowl and
blend with a hand-held stick blender to a purée (alternatively, blend
the mixture using a mini food processor). Stir in the remaining oil and
season to taste with salt and pepper.

Arrange the roasted tomatoes on a platter, then tear the mozzarella
balls in half and arrange the mozzarella chunks among the tomatoes.
Drizzle with the dressing and scatter with the pine nuts. Serve
immediately with gluten-free bread.

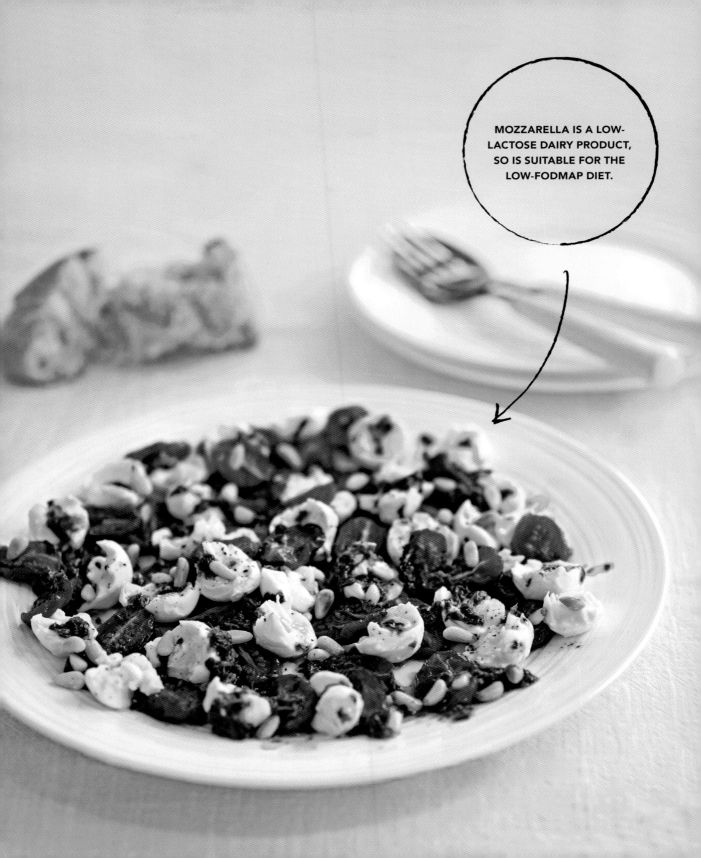

MOZZARELLA IS A LOW-LACTOSE DAIRY PRODUCT, SO IS SUITABLE FOR THE LOW-FODMAP DIET.

14oz white crabmeat

1 large orange, peeled
and sliced

1½ cups tightly packed
arugula

1 bunch of scallions
(green parts only), sliced

7oz steamed green snap
beans, sliced

salt and freshly ground
black pepper

FOR THE WATERCRESS DRESSING

3 cups watercress, tough stems
removed

1 tablespoon Dijon mustard

2 tablespoons olive oil

salt

TO SERVE

4 pieces gluten-free
pitta bread

lime wedges

CRAB & ORANGE SALAD

PREPARATION TIME: 15 MINUTES
COOKING TIME: 2 MINUTES
SERVES: 4

Combine the crabmeat, orange, arugula, scallions, and green snap beans in a serving dish. Season to taste with salt and pepper.

To make the dressing, put the watercress, mustard, and oil into the bowl of a food processor and blend together. Season with salt.

Toast the pitta bread. Stir the dressing into the salad and serve with the toasted pitta bread and lime wedges on the side.

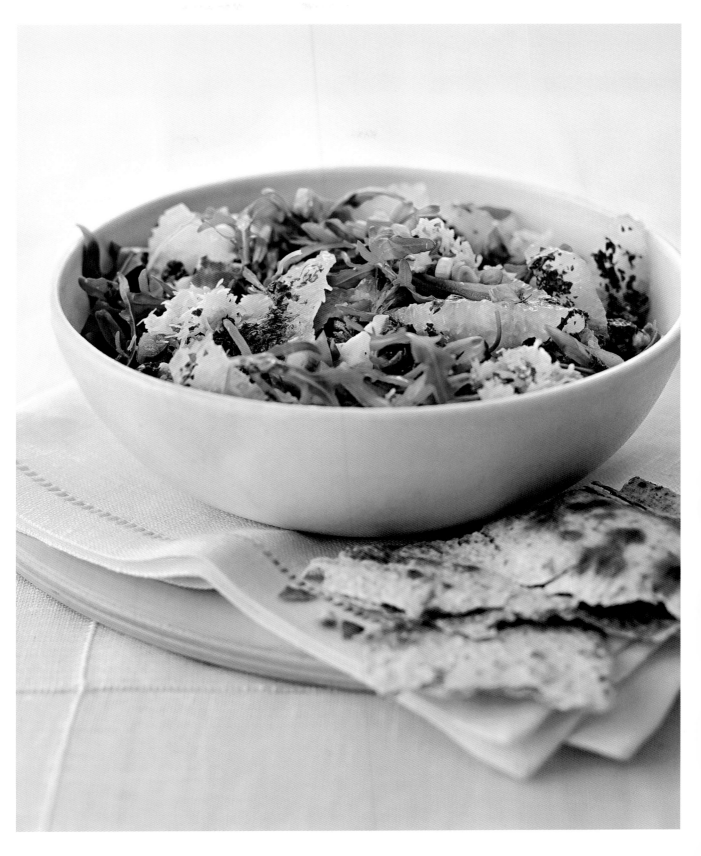

- 14oz new potatoes, halved
- 3 tablespoons olive oil, divided
- 2 teaspoons red wine vinegar
- 1 tablespoon wholegrain mustard
- 1 handful of chives, finely snipped
- 1 tablespoon rinsed and thinly sliced cornichons or gherkins (free from celery seeds)
- 2 teaspoons rinsed and drained capers
- 1 cup halved cherry tomatoes
- 2 tablespoons Kalamata olives, drained
- 4 small mackerel fillets, boned and skins lightly scored
- large handful of curly endive leaves
- salt and freshly ground black pepper

WARM POTATO & MACKEREL SALAD

PREPARATION TIME: 15 MINUTES, PLUS COOLING
COOKING TIME: 20 MINUTES
SERVES: 4

Cook the new potatoes in a large pan of salted boiling water for 12 to 15 minutes, until just tender. Drain the potatoes, return them to the pan, and toss with 2 tablespoons of the olive oil. Add the vinegar, mustard, chives, cornichons or gherkins, capers, tomatoes, and olives, then season to taste. Set aside.

Heat the remaining olive oil in a large, nonstick skillet and cook the mackerel fillets, skin-side down, for 3 to 4 minutes, or until the flesh turns white. Gently turn them over and cook for a further minute, until lightly golden. Remove from the pan and let cool slightly, then flake the flesh.

Arrange the curly endive on serving plates and serve with the warm potato salad and flaked mackerel.

2 teaspoons garlic-infused olive oil

1 teaspoon balsamic vinegar

4 small boneless, skinless chicken breasts, halved horizontally

FOR THE RICE SALAD

1 cup mixture of wild rice and basmati rice

2 red bell peppers, roasted, seeded, and sliced

3 scallions (green parts only), sliced

1 cup quartered cherry tomatoes

3 cups tighly packed arugula

2¾oz lactose-free soft goat cheese, crumbled

FOR THE DRESSING

2 tablespoons lemon juice

1 teaspoon Dijon mustard

1 teaspoon maple syrup

2 tablespoons olive oil

WILD RICE & GRIDDLED CHICKEN SALAD

PREPARATION TIME: 40 MINUTES, PLUS MARINATING
COOKING TIME: 35 MINUTES
SERVES: 4

Mix together the garlic-infused oil and vinegar in a nonmetallic bowl, add the chicken, and coat in the marinade. Cover and let marinate in the refrigerator for at least 30 minutes.

Cook the rice in a saucepan of boiling water following the package directions. Drain well and let cool, then mix with the bell peppers, scallions, tomatoes, arugula, and goat cheese in a large bowl.

Whisk together the dressing ingredients in another bowl. Stir the dressing into the rice salad. Spoon the salad onto 4 serving plates.

Heat a griddle until hot. Cook the chicken over medium-high heat for 3 to 4 minutes on each side, until cooked through. Just before serving, slice the griddled chicken and arrange it on top of the salad.

¼ cup olive oil, divided

1lb 10oz butternut squash, peeled, if liked, seeded, and cut into small chunks

13oz chicken livers

6oz bacon, cut into strips

1 cup walnuts

5½oz watercress

freshly ground black pepper

balsamic vinegar, to serve

LIMIT BALSAMIC VINEGAR TO 1 TABLESPOON PER SITTING ON THE LOW-FODMAP DIET.

WARM CHICKEN LIVER, BUTTERNUT SQUASH & BACON SALAD

PREPARATION TIME: 10 MINUTES, PLUS COOLING

COOKING TIME: 20 MINUTES

SERVES: 4

Heat 3 tablespoons of the oil in a large, heavy skillet or wok and cook the squash, stirring occasionally, over medium-high heat for 15 to 20 minutes, until softened and cooked through.

Meanwhile, in a separate heavy skillet, heat the remaining oil and cook the chicken livers and bacon over high heat for 10 minutes or until golden and cooked through, stirring almost continuously to stop them from sticking to the pan. Add the walnuts and cook for a further minute to warm through.

Toss together the chicken livers, bacon, walnuts, and squash in a large bowl, season with pepper, and set aside to cool for 3 to 4 minutes.

Just before serving, add the watercress to the bowl and toss to combine. Arrange the salad on 4 warmed serving plates and drizzle with balsamic vinegar.

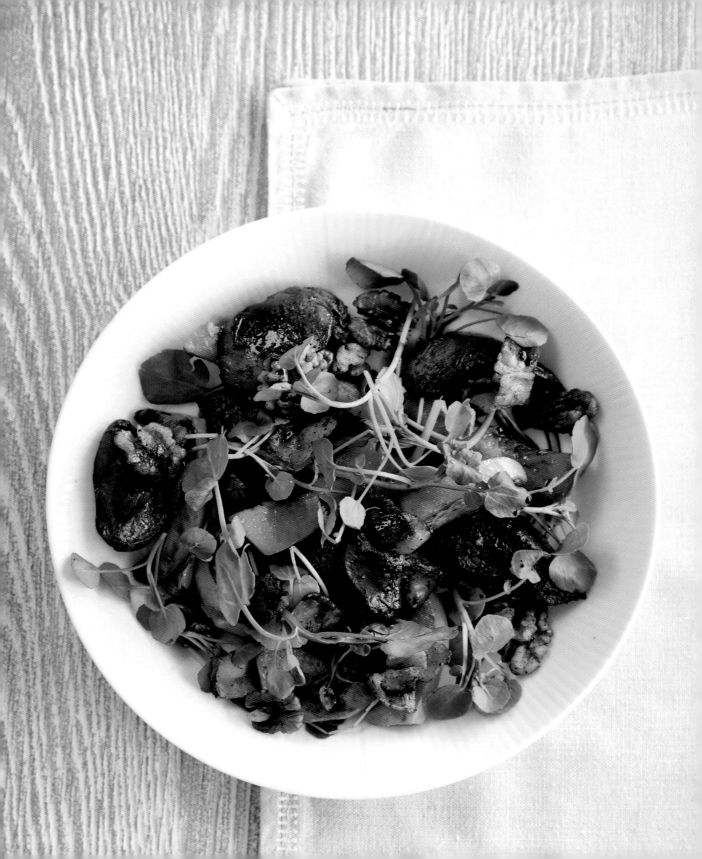

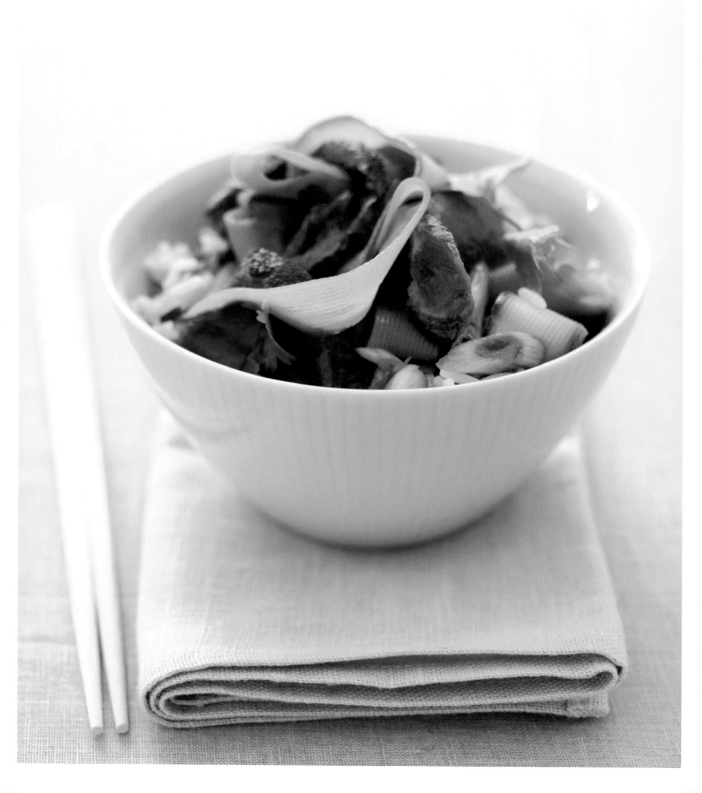

MARINATED THAI BEEF SALAD

PREPARATION TIME: 25 MINUTES
COOKING TIME: 20 TO 25 MINUTES
SERVES: 4

¾ cup mixture of long-grain rice and wild rice

finely grated zest and juice of 2 limes

1½lb thick-cut sirloin or porterhouse steak

2 tablespoons sesame oil

2 zucchini, cut into long, thin slices with a vegetable peeler

2 carrots, cut into long, thin slices with a vegetable peeler

4 scallions (green parts only), thinly sliced

1 large mild red chile, seeded and chopped

1½-inch piece of fresh ginger root, peeled and cut into thin strips

2 tablespoons soy sauce

¼ cup dry sherry or water

1 tablespoon Thai fish sauce

2 teaspoons superfine sugar

small bunch of fresh cilantro or mint, coarsely torn

Cook the rice in a saucepan of boiling water for 15 to 18 minutes or until just tender. Drain the cooked rice, rinse it in cold water, then drain thoroughly. Put the rice into a bowl with the lime zest and juice and toss together. Cover the bowl and place in the refrigerator.

Heat a skillet over high heat. Brush the steaks with the sesame oil, then cook them in the hot skillet over high heat for 1 to 3 minutes on each side, depending on how rare or well done you like your steak. Transfer to a shallow nonmetallic dish.

Put the zucchini and carrot strips into the hot skillet you used to cook the steaks. Add the scallions, chile, and ginger and fry briefly for 30 seconds. Transfer to the dish with the steak. Add the soy sauce, sherry or water, fish sauce, and sugar to the pan and warm gently. Pour the mixture over the steak and vegetables and let marinate and cool, then chill until required.

When ready to serve, transfer the rice to a salad bowl. Add the vegetables and sauce and the torn herbs and toss to combine. Cut the steak into thin slices and arrange on top of the rice salad.

1/3 cup extra-virgin olive oil, divided

14oz very fresh tuna steak

1 tablespoon black peppercorns, coarsely crushed

1 tablespoon balsamic vinegar

2 3/4 cups tightly packed wild arugula

salt

shavings of Parmesan cheese, to serve

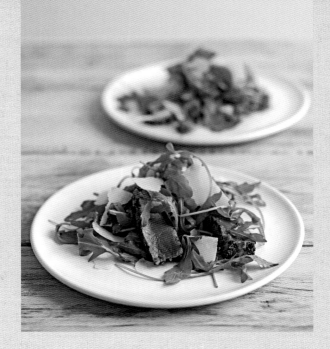

PEPPERED TUNA
WITH ARUGULA & PARMESAN

PREPARATION TIME: 10 MINUTES, PLUS COOLING
COOKING TIME: 10 MINUTES
SERVES: 4

Brush 1 tablespoon of the oil over the tuna. Place the crushed peppercorns on a plate, then roll the tuna in the pepper until well coated. Wrap up the tuna tightly in a piece of aluminum foil.

Heat a dry, heavy skillet until smoking hot. Add the wrapped tuna to the pan and cook for 7 minutes, turning every minute or so to cook evenly on each side. Remove from the pan and let cool a little.

Whisk the remaining oil with the vinegar until well combined, then season with salt.

Just before serving, unwrap the tuna and slice it. Toss the arugula with the dressing and arrange it on serving plates. Scatter with the tuna slices and Parmesan shavings to serve.

14oz gluten-free pasta

5½oz green snap beans, trimmed

7oz can tuna in springwater, drained and flaked

²⁄₃ cup quartered cherry tomatoes

½ cup pitted black olives

2¼ cups tightly packed arugula

salt

FOR THE DRESSING

3 anchovy fillets in oil, drained and chopped

2 teaspoons white wine vinegar

2 tablespoons garlic-infused olive oil

ENSURE THAT GARLIC-INFUSED OIL IS STRAINED WELL AND CONTAINS NO VISIBLE GARLIC RESIDUE.

PASTA NIÇOISE

PREPARATION TIME: 10 MINUTES
COOKING TIME: 10 MINUTES
SERVES: 4

Cook the pasta in a large saucepan of salted boiling water following the package directions until al dente, adding the beans 5 minutes before the end of the cooking time and cooking until the beans are just tender.

Meanwhile, make the dressing. Mash the anchovies in a bowl, then blend in the vinegar and oils.

Drain the pasta and beans, reserving a little of the cooking water. Return the mixture to the pan and stir through the dressing, adding just enough of the reserved cooking water to loosen, if needed. Stir through the remaining ingredients and serve immediately.

8 slices of day-old gluten-free bread, cut into bite-sized pieces

⅓ cup olive oil, divided

4 eggs

1 tablespoon Dijon mustard

2 tablespoons lemon juice

3½oz bacon, cut into bite-sized pieces

2¾ cups tightly packed arugula

salt and freshly ground black pepper

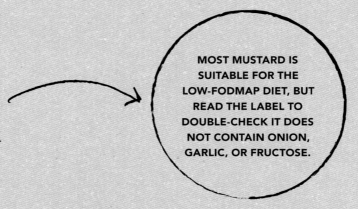

MOST MUSTARD IS SUITABLE FOR THE LOW-FODMAP DIET, BUT READ THE LABEL TO DOUBLE-CHECK IT DOES NOT CONTAIN ONION, GARLIC, OR FRUCTOSE.

SOFT-BOILED EGG & BACON SALAD

PREPARATION TIME: 10 MINUTES
COOKING TIME: 10 MINUTES
SERVES: 4

Preheat the oven to 400°F.

Put the bread into a bowl, add 2 tablespoons of the oil, and toss to coat. Spread out the pieces of bread on a baking pan and bake for 10 minutes or until golden brown.

Meanwhile, cook the eggs in a saucepan of boiling water for 4 minutes. Drain, then cool them under cold running water for 1 minute.

Whisk together the remaining oil, the mustard, and lemon juice in a small bowl.

Heat a nonstick skillet, add the bacon, and cook over medium heat for 5 minutes, until crisp and golden. Add the bacon pieces to a bowl along with the arugula.

Peel the eggs, then break them in half and add them to the bacon and arugula. Scatter the salad with the croûtons, then drizzle with the dressing. Season to taste and serve immediately.

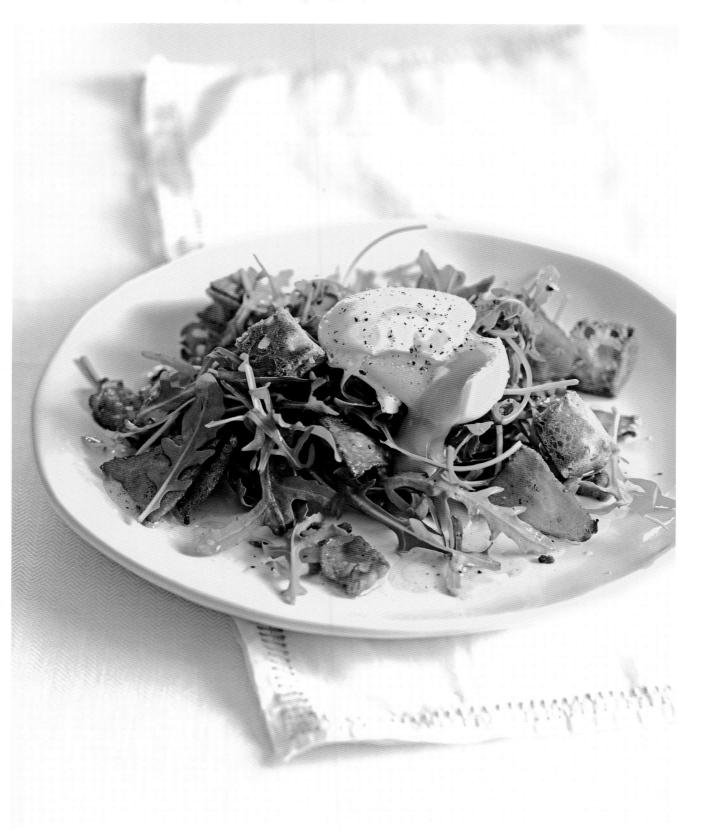

APPETIZERS & LIGHT BITES

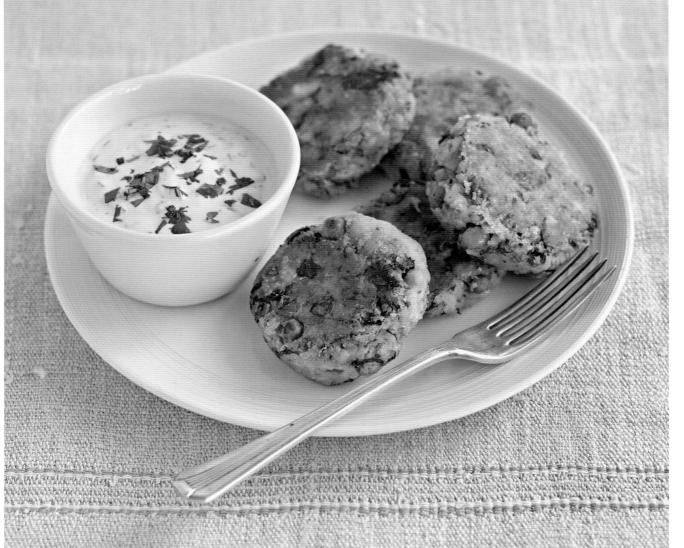

WHEN USING GARAM MASALA, CHECK TO ENSURE YOUR PRODUCT DOES NOT CONTAIN FODMAPS SUCH AS ONION AND GARLIC.

1½lb potatoes, peeled and cut into chunks

2 tablespoons chopped fresh cilantro

2 teaspoons peeled and finely grated fresh ginger root

2½ teaspoons garam masala

1 mild green chile, seeded and chopped

3½oz frozen spinach, defrosted

¾ cup fresh gluten-free bread crumbs

2 to 3 tablespoons gluten-free all-purpose flour

vegetable oil, for shallow-frying

salt and freshly ground black pepper

FOR THE CHUTNEY

2 tablespoons chopped fresh cilantro

2 tablespoons chopped mint

1 cup plain lactose-free or plant-based yogurt (limit soy yogurt to ¼ cup per portion), or standard yogurt if you know you tolerate lactose

2 teaspoons lemon juice

salt and freshly ground black pepper

ALOO TIKKI
WITH CILANTRO & MINT CHUTNEY

PREPARATION TIME: 20 MINUTES
COOKING TIME: 25 MINUTES
SERVES: 4

Cook the potatoes in a large saucepan of lightly salted boiling water for about 10 minutes or until just tender. Drain well.

Meanwhile, mix the cilantro with the grated ginger, garam masala, and chopped chile in a bowl.

Place the spinach in the middle of a clean dish cloth, bring up the edges and twist the spinach in the cloth over a sink to squeeze out excess moisture. Add to the bowl of spices, season generously with salt and pepper, and mix well to combine. Set aside.

To make the chutney, mix the cilantro with the mint, yogurt, and lemon juice. Season to taste, then set aside.

Add the potatoes to the spinach and mash well to combine. Add the bread crumbs and mix thoroughly to form a soft dough mixture. Form the mixture into 20 to 24 small patties and dust with the flour.

Heat the oil in a large skillet. Shallow-fry the patties over medium heat for 3 to 4 minutes, turning once, until crisp and golden. Drain on paper towels, then serve hot with the chutney.

PREPARATION TIME: 20 MINUTES
COOKING TIME: 20 MINUTES
SERVES: 4

1lb potatoes, peeled and diced

3 tablespoons olive oil, divided

1lb 2oz skinless salmon fillet

1 tablespoon chopped dill

finely grated zest of 1 lemon

gluten-free all-purpose flour, for dusting

1 egg, beaten

¾ cup dried gluten-free bread crumbs

salt and freshly ground black pepper

green salad, to serve

FOR THE DILL SAUCE

3 tablespoons mayonnaise (free from garlic and onion)

3 tablespoons plain lactose-free or plant-based yogurt (limit soy yogurt to ¼ cup per portion), or standard yogurt if you know you tolerate lactose

handful of dill, chopped

1 cornichon, sliced

SALMON FISHCAKES
WITH DILL SAUCE

Preheat the broiler on the highest setting.

Cook the potatoes in a saucepan of lightly salted boiling water for 12 minutes, until soft. Drain well and coarsely mash them.

Meanwhile, rub 1 teaspoon of the oil over the salmon and season well. Transfer to a roasting pan and broil for 10 minutes, until cooked through. Let cool a little, then break the flesh into large flakes.

Combine the sauce ingredients in a bowl and mix well.

Mix together the mashed potatoes, salmon flakes, dill, and lemon zest in a large bowl. Lightly wet your hands, then shape the mixture into 8 fishcakes. Dust each fishcake with a little flour, dip it into the egg, and, finally, dip it into the bread crumbs until well coated.

Heat the remaining oil in a large, nonstick skillet. Cook the fishcakes for 3 to 4 minutes on each side, until golden and crisp. Serve with a green salad and the dill sauce.

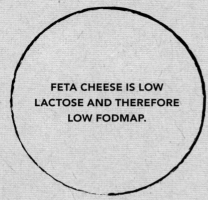

FETA CHEESE IS LOW LACTOSE AND THEREFORE LOW FODMAP.

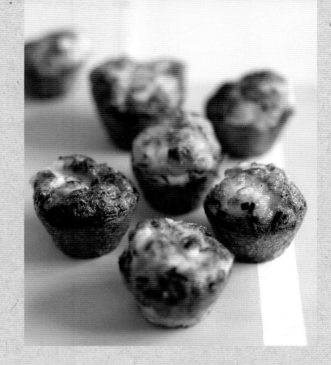

MINI TOMATO & FETA OMELETS

PREPARATION TIME: 10 MINUTES
COOKING TIME: 10 MINUTES
MAKES: 12

canola oil or vegetable oil, for greasing
....
4 eggs, beaten
....
2 tablespoons snipped chives
....
3 sun-dried tomatoes, finely sliced
....
½ cup crumbled feta cheese
....
salt and freshly ground black pepper

Preheat the oven to 425°F. Lightly grease a 12-hole mini muffin pan with oil.

Mix together all the ingredients in a large bowl until just combined. Pour the mixture into the prepared holes of the muffin pan.

Bake for about 10 minutes, until golden and puffed up. Transfer to a wire rack and let cool a little. Serve warm.

½ tablespoon canola oil

14oz baby spinach

6 large eggs

½ cup lactose-free or plant-based milk (limit soy to ¼ cup per portion), or standard milk if you know you tolerate lactose

3 tablespoons grated Parmesan cheese

2 tablespoons finely snipped chives

5½oz cooked hot-smoked trout or salmon fillets, flaked

4 cherry tomatoes, halved

salt and freshly ground black pepper

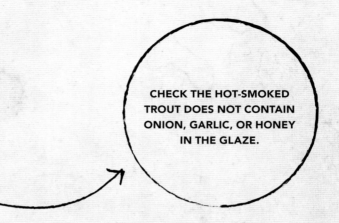

CHECK THE HOT-SMOKED TROUT DOES NOT CONTAIN ONION, GARLIC, OR HONEY IN THE GLAZE.

MINI SMOKED TROUT QUICHES

PREPARATION TIME: 15 MINUTES, PLUS COOLING

COOKING TIME: 20 MINUTES

SERVES: 4

Preheat the oven to 350°F. Line 8 holes of a muffin pan with 6-inch squares of nonstick parchment paper.

Heat the oil in a skillet, add the spinach, and cook briefly until wilted. Remove the pan from the heat.

Beat together the eggs, milk, and cheese in a large measuring cup and season to taste, then stir in the chives and trout or salmon.

Divide the spinach among the parchment-paper lined muffin pan holes, then pour in the egg mixture. Top each one with a tomato half. Bake for 12 to 15 minutes, until just set. Transfer to a wire rack and let cool a little. Serve warm or cold.

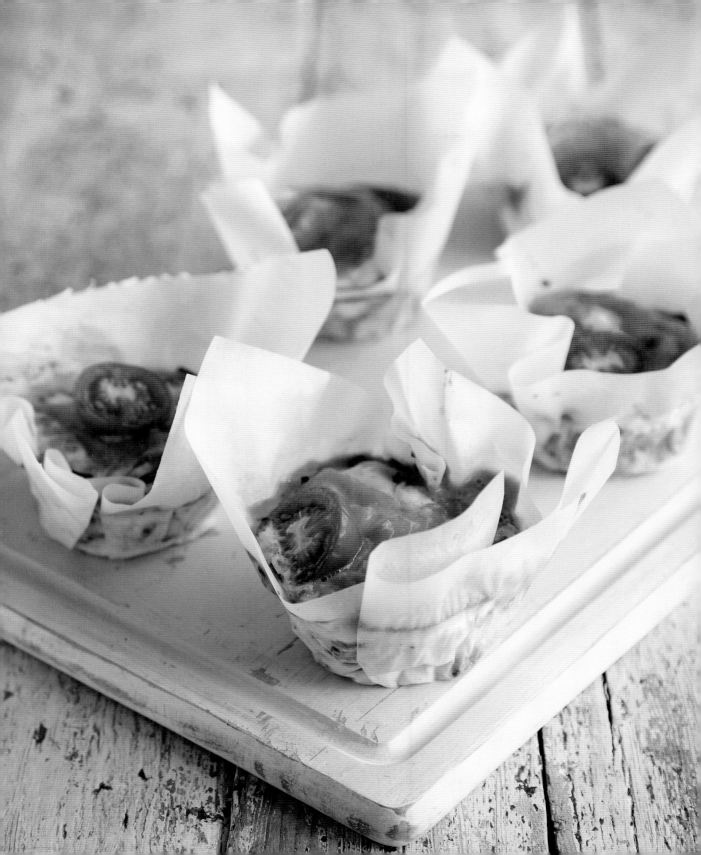

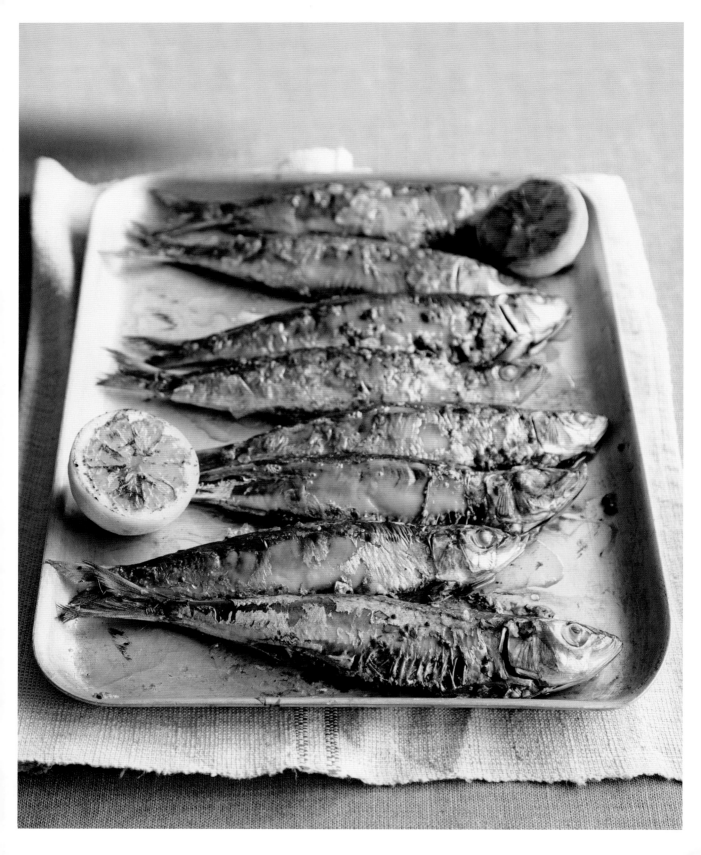

small handful of flat-leaf
parsley leaves, chopped

1 tablespoon wholegrain
mustard

¼ cup lemon juice

8 sardines, boned, cleaned
and gutted

2 tablespoons olive oil

lemon halves, to serve

SARDINES ARE AN OILY FISH, RICH IN OMEGA 3 FATS, WHICH ARE GREAT FOR THEIR BRAIN-BOOSTING POWER AND CARDIO-PROTECTIVE EFFECTS.

BROILED SARDINES
WITH LEMON & MUSTARD

PREPARATION TIME: 15 MINUTES
COOKING TIME: 10 MINUTES
SERVES: 4

Preheat the broiler on the highest setting.

Mix together the parsley, mustard, and lemon juice in a bowl, then spoon the mixture into the sardine cavities. Brush the fish with the oil.

Cook under the hot broiler for 4 minutes on each side or until cooked through. Serve with lemon halves.

PREPARATION TIME:

25 MINUTES, PLUS SOAKING
AND MARINATING

COOKING TIME: 25 MINUTES

SERVES: 4

3 dried ancho chiles, trimmed
and seeded

3 cloves

1/2 teaspoon cumin seeds

1/2 cinnamon stick

2 teaspoons dried oregano

1 tablespoon red wine vinegar

2 teaspoons maple syrup

1 tablespoon garlic-infused
olive oil

2 small pork tenderloins,
about 10½oz each
(or 1 large tenderloin,
about 1¼ lb)

salt and freshly ground
black pepper

FOR THE SALSA

1/2 ripe pineapple, peeled,
cored, and chopped

1 tablespoon finely chopped
scallions (green parts only)

1 red chile, seeded,
if liked, and chopped

juice of 1/2 lime

handful of fresh cilantro
leaves, chopped

salt and freshly ground
black pepper

SPICED PORK WITH PINEAPPLE SALSA

Heat a dry nonstick skillet until hot. Add the chiles and dry-fry for 1 minute on each side, until lightly toasted. Transfer to a heatproof bowl, pour in enough boiling water to cover, and let soak for 30 minutes until softened.

Add the whole spices to the same skillet you used to cook the chiles and cook over high heat for 30 seconds, until they release their aromas. Tip the mixture into a spice grinder (or use a mortar and pestle) and pound until finely ground.

Remove the chiles from the soaking liquid and put them into a mini processor or blender with the ground spices, oregano, vinegar, maple syrup, and oil and whizz to a smooth paste. Rub the mixture all

over the pork in a shallow nonmetallic dish. Cover the dish with plastic wrap and let marinate in the refrigerator for 2 hours.

Preheat the oven to 400°F.

Wipe any excess marinade off of the pork, then place it in a shallow roasting pan and season. Bake for 25 minutes, until just cooked through.

Meanwhile, make the salsa. Combine all the ingredients in a bowl. Season and mix well.

Cut the pork into thick slices and serve with the salsa.

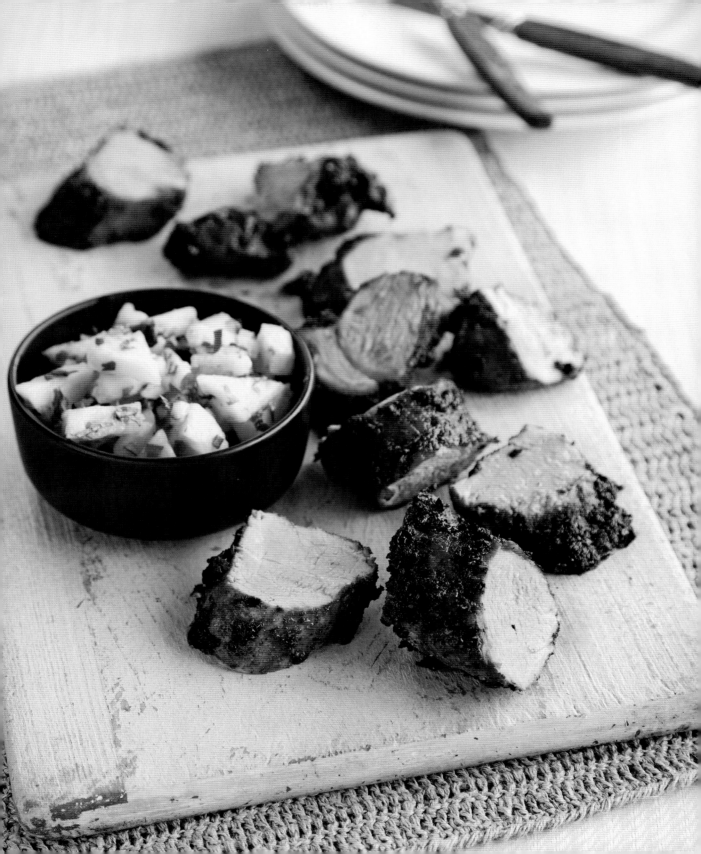

24 raw peeled jumbo shrimp, deveined

FOR THE MARINADE

¼ cup garlic-infused olive oil

2 teaspoons peeled and grated fresh ginger root

1 bird's-eye chile, seeded and sliced

4 kaffir lime leaves, torn

1 lemongrass stalk, finely sliced

2 tablespoons Thai fish sauce

2 tablespoons lime juice

4 teaspoons soft light brown sugar

salt and freshly ground black pepper

TO GARNISH

1 tablespoon each chopped fresh cilantro, mint, and Thai basil leaves

1 large red chile, seeded and sliced

SHRIMP WITH ASIAN DRESSING

PREPARATION TIME: 10 MINUTES, PLUS MARINATING
COOKING TIME: 6 MINUTES
SERVES: 4

Combine the marinade ingredients in a nonmetallic dish. Add the shrimp and stir well, then let marinate for 30 minutes. Meanwhile, soak 24 bamboo skewers in cold water for 30 minutes.

Thread 1 shrimp onto each skewer and tip the marinade juices into a small saucepan.

Cook the shrimp on a hot barbecue or ridged griddle pan for 2 minutes on each side, then arrange on a platter.

Meanwhile, bring the marinade juices to a boil, then drizzle the shrimp with them. Serve garnished with the herbs and chile slices.

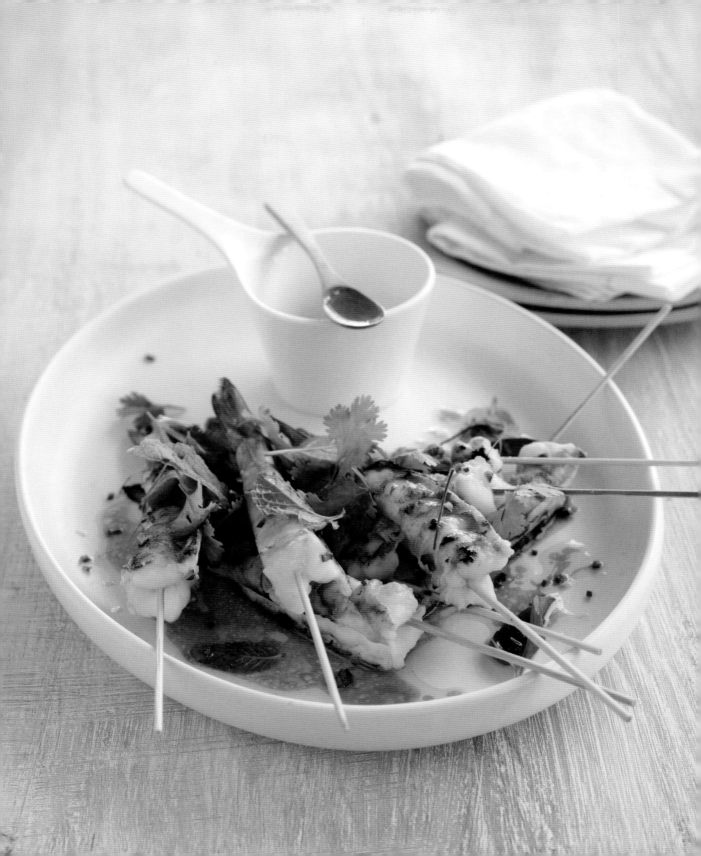

8 chicken drumsticks

2 tablespoons maple syrup

2 tablespoons olive oil

2 tablespoons dark soy sauce

1 teaspoon tomato paste

1 tablespoon Dijon mustard

chopped flat-leaf parsley,
to garnish

TO SERVE (OPTIONAL)

steamed rice

crisp green salad

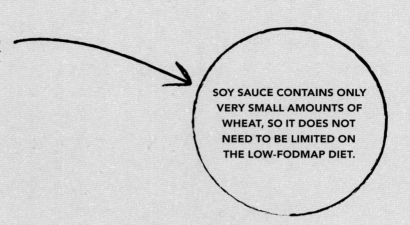

SOY SAUCE CONTAINS ONLY
VERY SMALL AMOUNTS OF
WHEAT, SO IT DOES NOT
NEED TO BE LIMITED ON
THE LOW-FODMAP DIET.

STICKY SOY-GLAZED DRUMSTICKS

PREPARATION TIME: 20 MINUTES
COOKING TIME: 30 MINUTES
SERVES: 4

Preheat the oven to 425°F.

Put the drumsticks onto a cutting board and make 4 deep slashes in each one along the thick part of the meat, cutting down to the bone on both sides.

Mix together the maple syrup, oil, soy sauce, tomato paste, and mustard in a large bowl. Toss the drumsticks in the glaze, turning to coat the meat well.

Transfer the drumsticks to a roasting pan and roast at the top of the oven for 20 to 25 minutes or until the chicken is cooked through. Garnish with parsley and serve with steamed rice and a crisp green salad, if liked.

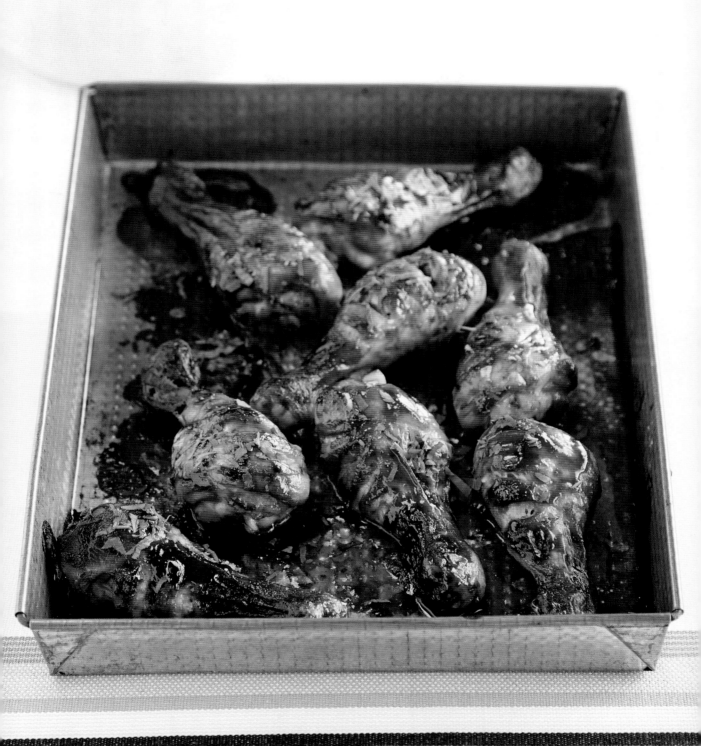

½ cup soy sauce

3 tablespoons smooth peanut butter (free from high-fructose corn syrup)

2 tablespoons water

2 chicken breasts, cut into strips

1 red bell pepper, seeded and cut into chunks

1 yellow bell pepper, seeded and cut into chunks

1 zucchini, halved and sliced

½ Napa cabbage, shredded

2 carrots, peeled and grated

¼ cup bean sprouts

small handful of fresh cilantro leaves

2 teaspoons sesame oil

juice of 1 lime

2 tablespoons sesame seeds, toasted, to serve

CHICKEN & VEGETABLE SATAY

PREPARATION TIME: 20 MINUTES
COOKING TIME: 15 MINUTES
SERVES: 4

Preheat the broiler on the highest setting. Soak 8 satay sticks in water.

Mix together the soy sauce, peanut butter, and measured water in a large bowl. Add the chicken, bell peppers, and zucchini pieces and toss them in the peanut butter mixture. Thread the chicken, bell peppers, and zucchini onto the soaked satay sticks.

Arrange the satay sticks on the pan of a broiler rack and broil for 12 to 14 minutes, turning regularly, until the chicken is cooked through.

Meanwhile, put the cabbage, grated carrot, bean sprouts, and cilantro leaves into a bowl with the sesame oil and lime juice and toss to coat.

Serve the satay with the salad, scattered with toasted sesame seeds.

- 6 thin slices of prosciutto
- 12 cleaned king scallops
- 4 long, sturdy stems of rosemary
- 3 tablespoons olive oil
- salt

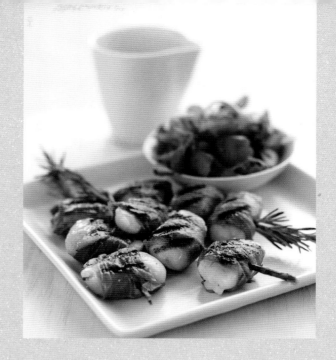

PROSCIUTTO, SCALLOP & ROSEMARY SKEWERS

PREPARATION TIME: 10 MINUTES
COOKING TIME: 5 MINUTES
SERVES: 4

Cut each slice of prosciutto in half lengthwise. Wrap one piece around each scallop.

Strip the leaves from the bottom of each rosemary stem, then thread 3 scallops onto each rosemary "skewer."

Drizzle the scallops with the oil and season with salt. Cook under a hot broiler or on a hot barbecue for 5 minutes, or until just cooked through, turning once.

2 lemongrass stalks

1 tablespoon garlic-infused oil

¼ cup peeled and sliced fresh ginger root

1 red chile

1 tablespoon soft light brown sugar, divided

¼ cup Thai fish sauce, divided

1lb 2oz beef steak strips

1 tablespoon oil

1¼lb fresh rice noodles

squeeze of lime juice

¼ iceberg lettuce, shredded

2 carrots, grated

handful of mint leaves

YOU CAN SUBSTITUTE 100 PERCENT BUCKWHEAT NOODLES FOR THE RICE NOODLES, SINCE THEY ARE ALSO LOW FODMAP.

GINGER BEEF SKEWERS

PREPARATION TIME: 15 MINUTES
COOKING TIME: 5 MINUTES
SERVES: 4

Put the lemongrass, garlic-infused oil, ginger, chile, half the sugar, and half the fish sauce into a blender and whizz to form a paste.

Rub the mixture all over the beef strips. Thread the meat onto skewers, then drizzle with the oil.

Heat a large ridged grill pan until smoking. Cook the meat skewers for 1 to 2 minutes on each side, until charred. Transfer to serving plates.

Meanwhile, cook the noodles following the package directions. Cool the noodles under cold running water and let drain.

Stir the remaining sugar and fish sauce together with the lime juice. Toss the mixture through the noodles along with the lettuce, carrots, and mint leaves and serve alongside the skewers.

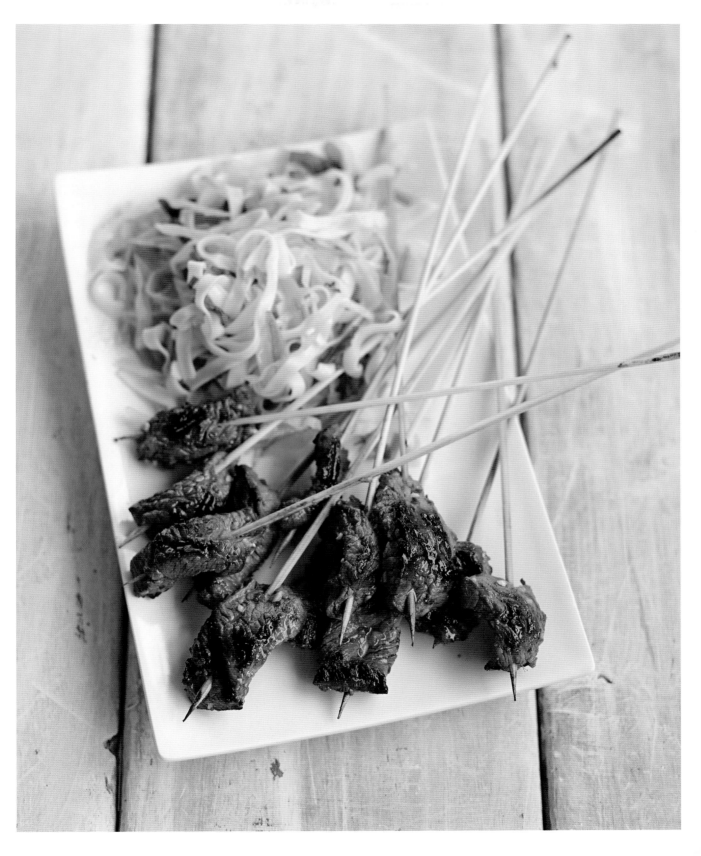

¾ cup gluten-free
all-purpose flour

1 teaspoon gluten-free
baking powder

½ teaspoon turmeric

2 teaspoons ground coriander

1 teaspoon ground cumin

1 teaspoon chili powder

1 cup soda water, chilled

sunflower oil, for deep-frying

1lb 6oz zucchini, cut into
thick batons

salt

plain lactose-free or
plant-based yogurt (limit soy
yogurt to ¼ cup per portion),
or standard yogurt if you
know you tolerate lactose

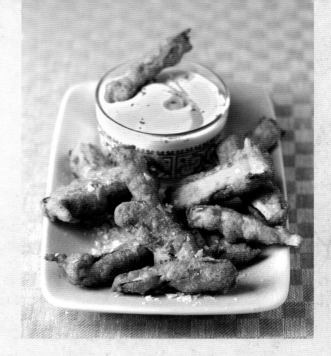

SPICED ZUCCHINI FRITTERS

PREPARATION TIME: 15 MINUTES
COOKING TIME: 10 MINUTES
SERVES: 4

Sift the flour, baking powder, turmeric, coriander, cumin, and chili powder into a large mixing bowl. Season with salt and gradually add the soda water to make a thick batter, being careful not to overmix.

Pour sunflower oil into a wok until it is one-third full. Heat the oil to 350 to 375°F, or until a cube of bread immersed in the oil browns in 30 seconds.

Dip the zucchini batons in the spiced batter, then deep-fry in batches for 1 to 2 minutes or until crisp and golden. Remove with a slotted spoon and drain on paper towels. Serve the zucchini batons immediately with the yogurt on the side for dipping.

- 8oz firm tofu
- 1 tablespoon light soy sauce
- 1 tablespoon oyster sauce
- 1 tablespoon sesame oil
- 3 tablespoons chopped fresh cilantro, divided
- 1 small red chile, seeded and finely chopped
- 1-inch piece of fresh ginger root, peeled and grated
- 2 teaspoons sesame seeds
- 1⅓ cups bean sprouts
- 2 scallions (green parts only), thinly sliced
- 1 tablespoon dark soy sauce

SILKEN TOFU IS HIGH IN FODMAPS AND SHOULD BE AVOIDED. FIRM TOFU IS FINE BECAUSE IT HAS A LOWER FODMAP CONTENT, BUT DISCARD THE WATER AS THIS IS THE PART THAT IS HIGHER IN FODMAPS.

ORIENTAL TOFU WITH SESAME SEEDS

PREPARATION TIME: 20 MINUTES, PLUS MARINATING
COOKING TIME: 5 MINUTES
SERVES: 4

Cut the tofu into 4 thin slices and add them to a bowl along with the light soy sauce, oyster sauce, sesame oil, 2 tablespoons of the chopped cilantro, the chile, and ginger and gently toss to mix. Cover the bowl with plastic wrap and marinate in the refrigerator for 2 hours or overnight.

Remove the tofu from the marinade and place it on a plate. Scatter both sides of the tofu slices with the sesame seeds.

Heat a griddle until hot. Set the tofu on the hot griddle and cook over medium heat for 1 to 2 minutes on each side, until scorched.

Toss the bean sprouts and scallions with the dark soy sauce in a bowl, then divide the mixture between 4 small plates. Top with the hot tofu and scatter with the remaining chopped cilantro. Serve as an appetizer.

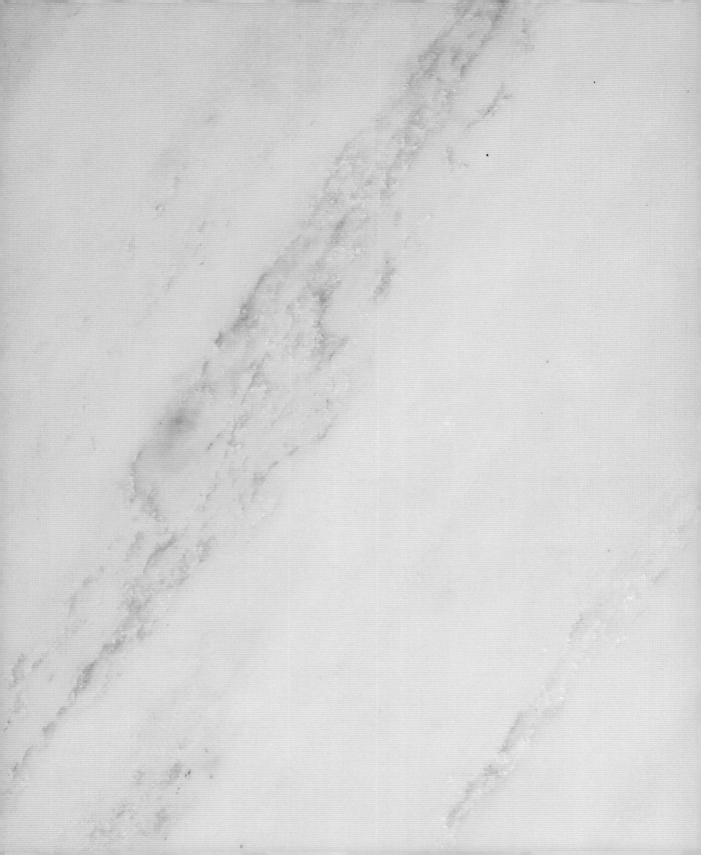

MAIN MEALS

pinch of saffron threads

1 tablespoon boiling water

4 skinless chicken drumsticks

4 skinless small chicken thighs

1 lemon, halved

2 tablespoons maple syrup

2/3 cup dry white wine

3/4 cup green olives

salt and freshly ground black pepper

2 tablespoons coarsely chopped flat-leaf parsley, to garnish

TO SERVE

cooked new potatoes

cooked green snap beans (limit each portion to 3oz)

CHICKEN ROASTED
WITH LEMON, OLIVES & SAFFRON

PREPARATION TIME: 15 MINUTES
COOKING TIME: 25 MINUTES
SERVES: 4

Preheat the oven to 425°F.

Soak the saffron threads in the measured boiling water in a small bowl.

Cut a couple of slashes across the top of each piece of chicken and season with salt and pepper. Spread out the chicken in a large roasting pan or ovenproof dish and squeeze the juice from the lemon halves over them. Drizzle with the maple syrup, pour the saffron threads and soaking water over them, and add the white wine. Roast for 20 minutes, basting with the juices occasionally. Add the olives and cook for a further 5 minutes, until the chicken is cooked through.

Scatter with the chopped parsley and serve with new potatoes and green snap beans.

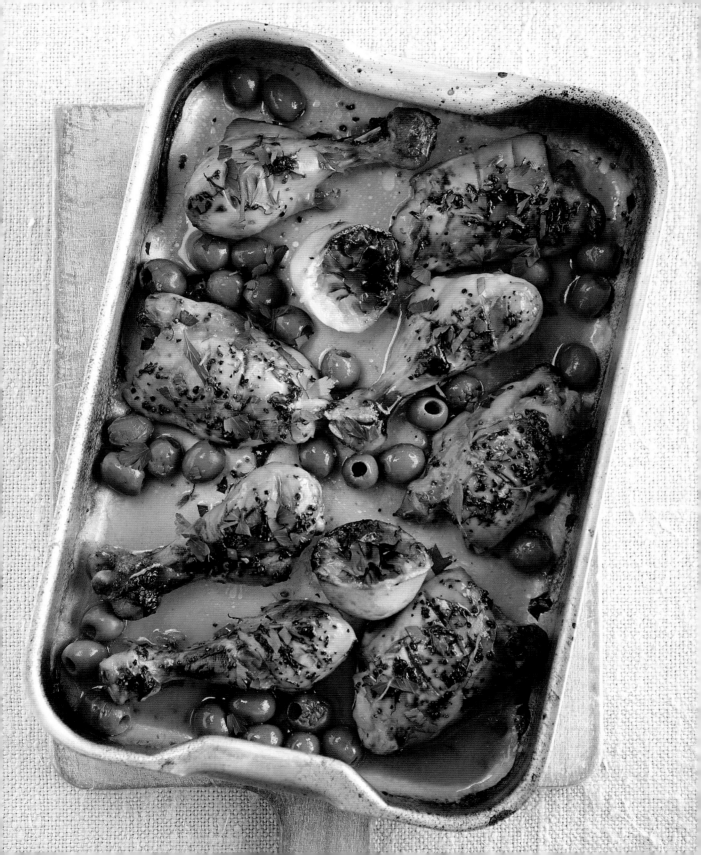

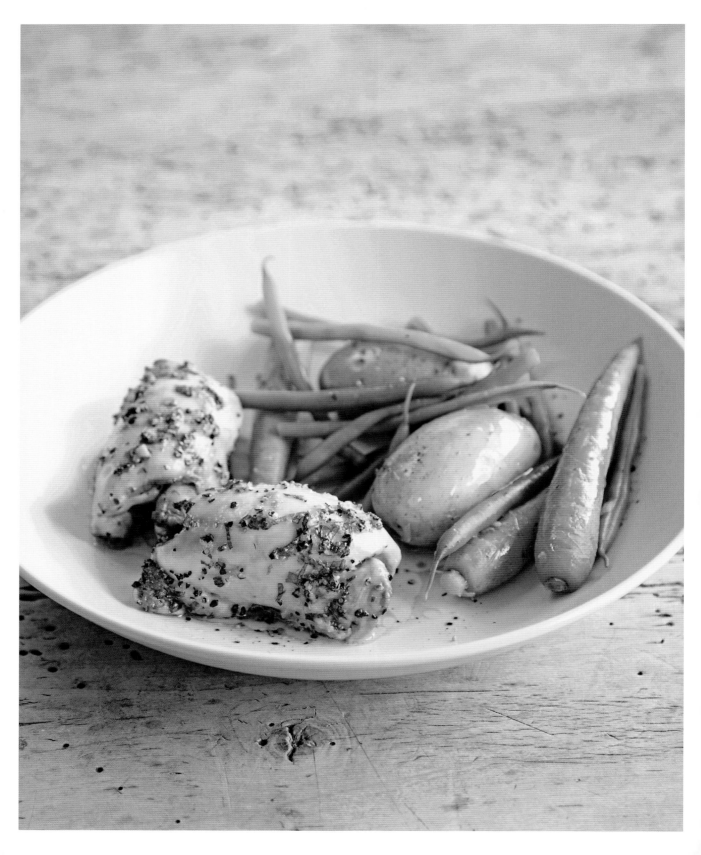

8 boneless, skinless chicken thighs

finely grated zest and juice of 1 lemon

3 tablespoons chopped flat-leaf parsley

½ stick butter

freshly ground black pepper

cooked seasonal vegetables, to serve

BUTTER, THOUGH MADE FROM MILK, IS NATURALLY LOW FODMAP AS IT IS VERY LOW IN LACTOSE. THIS MEANS YOU DON'T NEED TO BUY SPECIAL LOW-LACTOSE BUTTER.

CHICKEN THIGHS ROASTED
WITH BUTTER & LEMON

PREPARATION TIME: 10 MINUTES
COOKING TIME: 20 TO 25 MINUTES
SERVES: 4

Preheat the oven to 400°F.

Put the chicken thighs into a large bowl with the lemon zest and juice, parsley, and plenty of pepper and mix well to coat the chicken. Roll each of the coated thighs back into shape and secure each with a wooden toothpick.

Put the chicken thighs into a roasting pan, pouring any remaining juices over them, and top each with a small lump of butter. Roast for 20 to 25 minutes, or until golden and cooked through. Serve with seasonal vegetables.

4 lamb loin chops,
about 7oz each

1 tablespoon extra-virgin
olive oil

1½ tablespoons dried oregano

salt and freshly ground black
pepper

arugula, to garnish

FOR THE OLIVE & PINE NUT SALSA

3 tablespoons extra-virgin
olive oil, divided

2 tablespoons pine nuts,
toasted

1 cup pitted black olives,
halved

2 tablespoons drained capers
in brine

2 tablespoons chopped flat-leaf
parsley

1 tablespoon lemon juice

salt and freshly ground black
pepper

LAMB
WITH OLIVE & PINE NUT SALSA

**PREPARATION TIME: 10 MINUTES,
        PLUS COOLING**
COOKING TIME: 10 MINUTES
SERVES: 4

Make the salsa. Heat 1 tablespoon of the oil in a small skillet over low heat, add the pine nuts, and cook gently for 30 seconds until golden. Let cool.

Combine the cooled pine nuts with the olives, capers, parsley, lemon juice, and remaining oil in a bowl and season to taste with salt and pepper.

Heat a griddle until hot. Meanwhile, brush the chops with the oil and season with the oregano and salt and pepper. Transfer the chops to the hot griddle and cook over medium-high heat for 4 minutes on each side, until cooked.

Remove the chops from the pan, wrap loosely in aluminum foil, and let rest for 5 minutes. Serve garnished with the arugula, with the salsa on the side.

4 eggplants

10½oz ground lamb

2 pinches of ground cinnamon

1 tablespoon garlic-infused olive oil

½ cup cooked long-grain rice

2 tablespoons pine nuts

1 bunch of scallions (green parts only), chopped

2 tablespoons finely chopped mint

2 tablespoons finely chopped flat-leaf parsley

salt and freshly ground black pepper

GARLIC-INFUSED OLIVE OIL IS LOW FODMAP BECAUSE THE FRUCTANS IN GARLIC ARE WATER-SOLUBLE AND THEREFORE DO NOT ENTER INTO THE OIL, SO YOU GET ALL THE GARLIC TASTE WITH NONE OF THE FODMAPS.

EGGPLANTS STUFFED
WITH LAMB

PREPARATION TIME: 15 MINUTES
COOKING TIME: 35 MINUTES
SERVES: 4

Preheat the oven to 350°F.

Rinse and dry the eggplants, then halve them lengthwise and hollow out some of the flesh with a small spoon. Place the hollowed-out eggplants on a baking pan and bake for approximately 10 minutes, until slightly softened.

Season the ground lamb with the cinnamon and add salt and pepper to taste.

Heat the oil in a nonstick saucepan. Add the lamb, rice, pine nuts, scallion, and chopped mint and parsley and mix well. Cook for 8 to 10 minutes, until the lamb is browned and the liquid has evaporated.

Fill the hollowed-out eggplants with the lamb mixture. Return the eggplants to the oven and bake for 15 minutes or until piping hot. If necessary, add a little water in the bottom of the dish to ensure the eggplants do not stick. Serve warm or cold.

EGGPLANT & HARISSA SAUTÉ

PREPARATION TIME: 15 MINUTES
COOKING TIME: 10 MINUTES
SERVES: 4

¼ cup sunflower oil

1½lb baby eggplants, thinly sliced

4 tomatoes, chopped

1 teaspoon ground cinnamon

1 teaspoon finely chopped fresh cilantro leaves

2 tablespoons Low-FODMAP Harissa Paste (see below)

salt and freshly ground black pepper

cooked basmati rice, to serve

Heat the oil in a large skillet over high heat and add the eggplant slices. Fry for 2 to 3 minutes, then add the tomatoes, cinnamon, cilantro, and harissa. Stir-fry for 3 to 4 minutes, or until the eggplant slices are tender.

Season to taste and serve with basmati rice.

LOW-FODMAP HARISSA PASTE

Ready-made harissa paste contains garlic and is off-limits for those following the low-FODMAP diet. This homemade alternative is delicious and easy to make.

In advance of making the paste, soak 8 to 10 dried red chiles in water for 2 days. To make the paste, dry-fry 2 teaspoons each of cumin and cilantro seeds in a heavy skillet over medium heat for 2 to 3 minutes, until they release a nutty aroma, then grind them to a powder using a mortar and pestle. Drain the chiles, chop off the stems, and squeeze out most of the seeds. Discard the stems and seeds and coarsely chop the chiles. Pound the chiles with 1 to 2 teaspoons of sea salt using a mortar and pestle. Add the ground spices and pound again, then beat in 3 tablespoons of garlic-infused olive oil. Transfer the paste to a sterilized jar and top off with another tablespoon of the oil. Seal securely and store in a cool place or in the refrigerator. Use within 2 months.

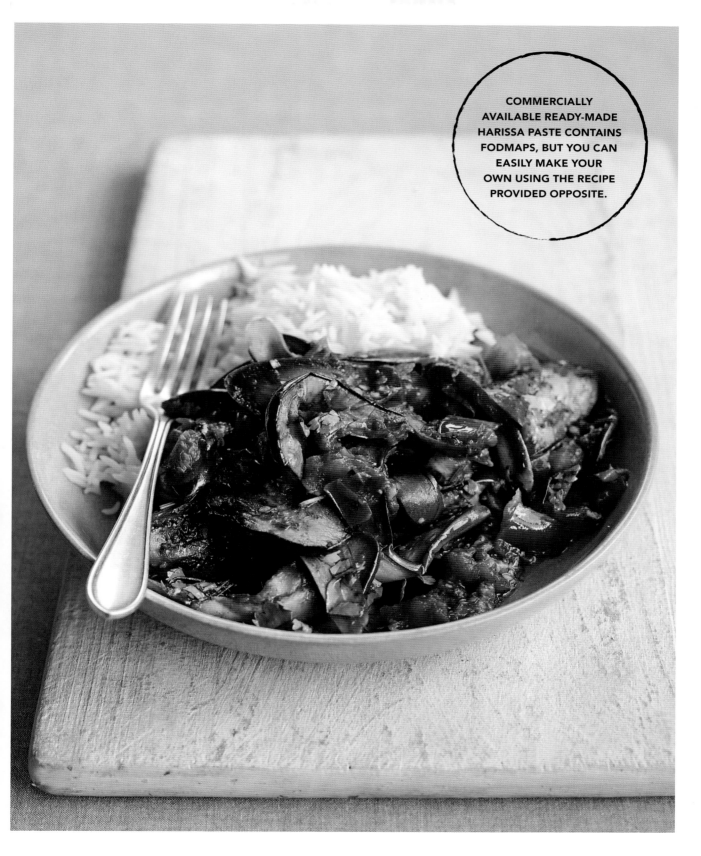

COMMERCIALLY AVAILABLE READY-MADE HARISSA PASTE CONTAINS FODMAPS, BUT YOU CAN EASILY MAKE YOUR OWN USING THE RECIPE PROVIDED OPPOSITE.

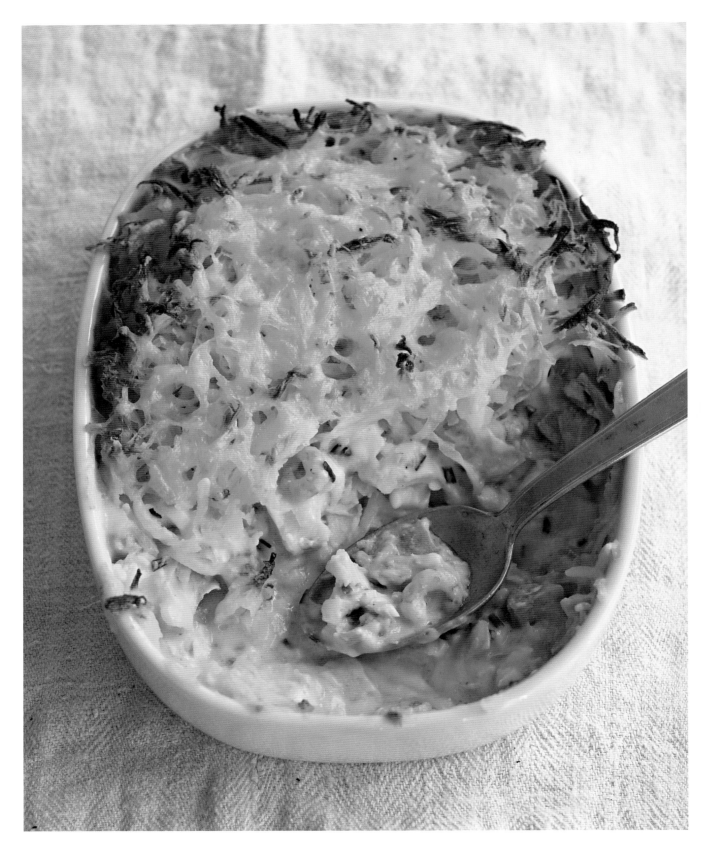

- 1lb 10oz potatoes, unpeeled
- 9oz white fish fillet (such as pollock or haddock), cut into bite-sized pieces
- 9oz salmon fillet, cut into bite-sized pieces
- 1¾ cups hot lactose-free or plant-based milk (limit soy to ¼ cup per portion), or standard milk if you know you tolerate lactose
- ½ stick butter
- ½ cup gluten-free flour
- 1 cup grated Cheddar cheese, divided
- 2 teaspoons lemon juice
- 2 tablespoons snipped chives
- 3½oz small cooked shelled shrimp (optional)
- salt and freshly ground black pepper

EASY FISH PIE
WITH CRUNCHY POTATO TOPPING

PREPARATION TIME: 20 MINUTES
COOKING TIME: 30 MINUTES
SERVES: 4

Preheat the oven to 350°F.

Cook the potatoes in a large saucepan of lightly salted water for 6 to 7 minutes. Drain and set aside to cool slightly.

Meanwhile, place the white fish and salmon in a deep-sided skillet. Pour in the hot milk and bring to a boil. Reduce the heat and let simmer gently for 3 to 4 minutes, until the fish is just cooked. Strain the milk into a pitcher and transfer the fish to an ovenproof dish.

Put the butter and flour into a saucepan and over very low heat to melt the butter. Stir for 2 minutes to cook the flour.

Add the reserved milk to the saucepan a little at a time, stirring well to incorporate it. Stir for a further 2 to 3 minutes, until thickened, then remove from the heat and stir in half the cheese, the lemon juice, and the chives, and season to taste. Pour the sauce over the fish, add the shrimp, if using, and stir gently to coat.

Wearing rubber gloves to protect your hands from the heat, grate the potatoes coarsely and scatter the grated potato over the fish. Scatter with the remaining cheese and bake for 15 to 20 minutes, or until the topping is golden and crispy.

3 tablespoons gluten-free
all-purpose flour

1 large egg, beaten

¼ cup gluten-free
bread crumbs

¼ cup polenta

1lb 2oz cod fillet, cut
into 8 thick pieces

3 tablespoons sunflower oil

GLUTEN-FREE FLOURS
AND BREAD CRUMBS ARE
RECOMMENDED BECAUSE
GLUTEN-FREE PRODUCTS
ARE GENERALLY WHEAT-
FREE AND THEREFORE
LOW FODMAP.

HOMEMADE FISH FINGERS

PREPARATION TIME: 10 MINUTES
COOKING TIME: 10 MINUTES
SERVES: 4

Put the flour and the beaten egg into 2 separate shallow bowls, then mix the bread crumbs and polenta together in a third bowl.

Gently toss the pieces of fish first in the flour, then in the egg, and finally in the bread crumb and polenta mixture to coat.

Heat the sunflower oil in a skillet over medium heat. Add the fish fingers carefully and cook for 5 to 6 minutes, turning occasionally, until golden. Drain on paper towels before serving.

1lb 6oz skinless haddock fillet

2½ cups lactose-free or plant-based milk (limit soy to ¼ cup per portion), or standard milk if you know you tolerate lactose

1 bay leaf

3 tablespoons butter

⅓ cup gluten-free all-purpose flour

½ cup grated Gruyère cheese

½ teaspoon English mustard

salad, to serve

FOR THE TOPPING

1 cup fresh gluten-free bread crumbs

¼ cup finely grated Gruyère cheese

finely grated zest of 1 lemon

2 tablespoons chopped flat-leaf parsley

CREAMY HADDOCK GRATIN

PREPARATION TIME: 10 MINUTES
COOKING TIME: 25 MINUTES
SERVES: 4

Preheat the oven to 425°F.

Place the haddock in a saucepan with the milk and bay leaf, bring to a boil, then let boil for 3 minutes. Remove the fish with a slotted spoon (reserve the milk), and divide it between 4 individual gratin dishes.

Melt the butter in a separate saucepan over medium heat, then add the flour, and cook, stirring, for a few seconds. Remove from the heat and add the reserved milk, a little at a time, stirring well between each addition. Return the pan to the heat, bring to a boil, and cook, stirring constantly, until thickened. Remove the pan from the heat and stir in the grated Gruyère and mustard to make a sauce.

Pour the sauce over the fish, dividing it evenly between the servings. Mix together all the ingredients for the topping and scatter the mixture over the sauce. Place the gratin dishes on the top rack in the oven and bake for 10 minutes, or until the topping is golden and the sauce is bubbling. Serve with a simple salad.

- 1 mild green chile, seeded and chopped
- 1 teaspoon ground coriander
- ½ teaspoon turmeric
- 1-inch piece of fresh ginger root, peeled and sliced
- 1 teaspoon garlic-infused oil
- 1 tablespoon coconut oil
- 1 bunch of scallions (green parts only), sliced
- 1 teaspoon cumin seeds
- ⅔ cup coconut milk
- 1 cup water
- 1lb mackerel fillets, cut into 2-inch pieces
- small handful of fresh cilantro leaves, coarsely torn
- salt and freshly ground black pepper
- cooked basmati rice, to serve

MACKEREL CURRY

PREPARATION TIME: 15 MINUTES
COOKING TIME: 20 MINUTES
SERVES: 4

Place the chile, ground coriander, turmeric, ginger, and garlic-infused oil in a small blender and blend to a smooth paste.

Heat the coconut oil in a wok or large skillet over medium heat. Add the spice paste, scallions, and cumin seeds and cook for 2 to 3 minutes, until the spices are fragrant.

Pour in the coconut milk and measured water. Bring to a boil, then simmer for 5 minutes. Season with salt and pepper.

Add the mackerel pieces to the wok or skillet and cook for 6 to 8 minutes, until the fish is cooked, then stir in the cilantro leaves. Serve immediately, with basmati rice, if liked.

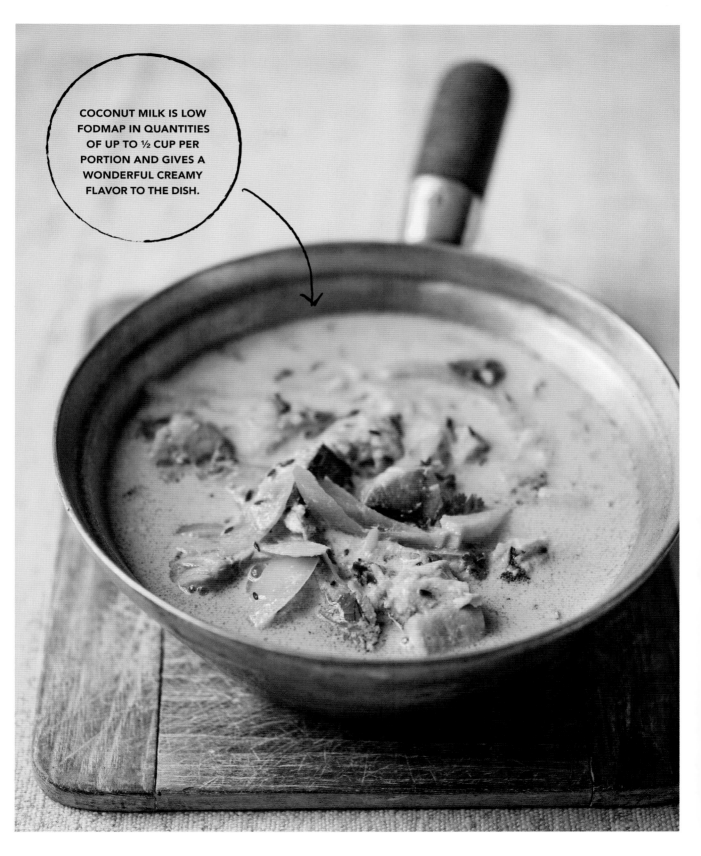

COCONUT MILK IS LOW FODMAP IN QUANTITIES OF UP TO ½ CUP PER PORTION AND GIVES A WONDERFUL CREAMY FLAVOR TO THE DISH.

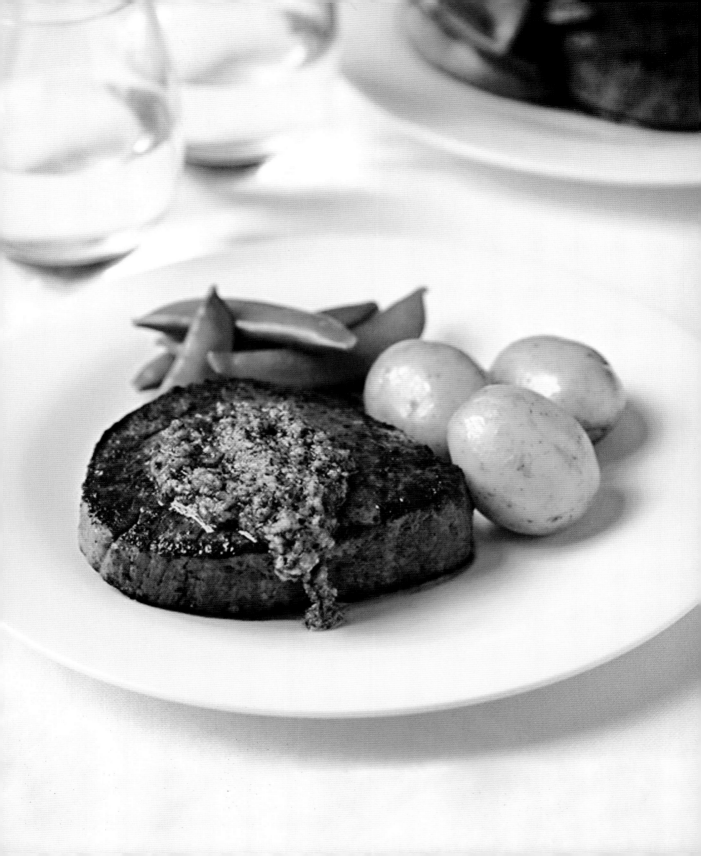

2 pieces of beef tenderloin,
about 7oz each

salt and freshly ground black
pepper

steamed new potatoes, to serve

FOR THE PESTO

½ cup toasted walnut halves

3 tablespoons chopped mixed
herbs (such as cilantro,
parsley, and basil)

2 tablespoons grated Parmesan
cheese

2 tablespoons garlic-infused
olive oil

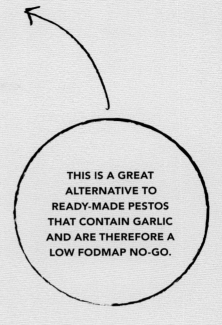

THIS IS A GREAT
ALTERNATIVE TO
READY-MADE PESTOS
THAT CONTAIN GARLIC
AND ARE THEREFORE A
LOW FODMAP NO-GO.

BEEF TENDERLOIN
WITH WALNUT PESTO

PREPARATION TIME: 20 MINUTES
COOKING TIME: 5 MINUTES
SERVES: 2

Heat a griddle or heavy skillet over high heat. Season the meat with
salt and pepper, add it to the pan, and cook for 2 minutes on each
side or until done to your liking.

Meanwhile, make the pesto. Put all the ingredients into the bowl
of a food processor or blender and process until combined but
still textured.

Serve the cooked steaks with the sauce drizzled on top, with
steamed new potatoes on the side.

BEEF WITH
HORSERADISH & QUINOA

PREPARATION TIME: 15 MINUTES, PLUS RESTING
COOKING TIME: 20 MINUTES
SERVES: 4

1lb 6oz beef tenderloin, rolled and tied

1 tablespoon horseradish sauce

2 tablespoons olive oil

1½ cups quinoa

1 green bell pepper, seeded and sliced

1 bunch of scallions (green parts only), thinly sliced

1 tablespoon chopped flat-leaf parsley

1 tablespoon chopped mint

1 cup tightly packed arugula

Preheat the oven to 400° F.

Brush the beef with the horseradish sauce.

Heat 1 tablespoon of the oil in a skillet over high heat. Add the beef and sear on all sides, until browned. Transfer the beef to a roasting pan and bake for 20 minutes, until done to your liking. Cover the pan with aluminum foil. Let rest for 5 to 6 minutes, then slice the beef.

Meanwhile, cook the quinoa in a saucepan of boiling water for 8 to 9 minutes, or following the package directions.

Heat the remaining oil in a large skillet over medium heat. Add the pepper and cook for 3 to 4 minutes until softened. Add the scallion and cook for a further minute. Remove the pan from the heat and stir in the chopped herbs.

Drain the quinoa and stir it into the peppers, scallion, and herbs. Divide the mixture between 4 warmed plates and top with the arugula and sliced beef.

1lb 2oz ground pork

2 scallions (green parts only), finely chopped, plus extra to garnish

1 tablespoon peeled and very finely chopped fresh ginger root

1 tablespoon cornstarch

1 small egg white, whisked

3 to 4 tablespoons vegetable or peanut oil

1¾ cups jasmine rice

salt

soy sauce, to serve (optional)

FOR THE SWEET & SOUR SAUCE

8oz can pineapple chunks in juice

½ cup tomato ketchup (free from fructose, onion and garlic)

2½ tablespoons soft light brown sugar

2 tablespoons malt vinegar

2 teaspoons light soy sauce

GROUND PORK BALLS
WITH SWEET & SOUR SAUCE

PREPARATION TIME: 15 MINUTES
COOKING TIME: 30 TO 40 MINUTES
SERVES: 4

Add the ground pork to a large bowl along with the scallions and ginger root. Whisk the cornstarch into the egg white and add it to the pork, stirring until well combined. Form the mixture into 20 to 24 balls.

Heat the oil in a large nonstick skillet over medium-high heat. Cook the meatballs for 10 to 12 minutes, until cooked through and golden.

Meanwhile, place the rice in a saucepan with 1½ times its volume of cold water. Bring to a boil, season with salt, cover the pan with a lid, and simmer gently for 11 to 14 minutes, or until the rice is tender and the liquid has been absorbed. Garnish with the extra scallions.

Make the sweet and sour sauce. Tip the pineapple and its juice into a mini-chopper or food processor and pulse until crushed but not smooth. (Or chop it finely by hand.) Pour the crushed pineapple into a small pan with the remaining ingredients and bring the mixture to a boil, then reduce the heat and simmer gently for 5 to 7 minutes, until thickened.

Drain the excess oil from the pan of meatballs, then pour the sauce into the pan and simmer for a 1 to 2 minutes, until the meatballs are well coated in the sauce. Spoon the meatballs and sauce over the rice and serve immediately with soy sauce, if desired.

2 tablespoons maple syrup

2 tablespoons dark soy sauce

2 teaspoons Chinese five-spice powder

1 teaspoon Szechuan pepper, lightly crushed

1 teaspoon peeled and finely grated fresh ginger root

2 teaspoons sesame oil, divided

1lb 2oz pork loin, thickly sliced

1 red bell pepper, seeded and thinly sliced

¾lb Napa cabbage, thinly sliced

2 cups bean sprouts

¾lb baby bok choy, halved lengthwise

2 teaspoons sesame seeds, to serve

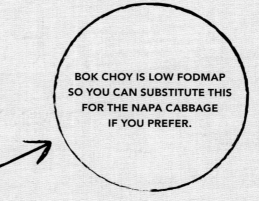

BOK CHOY IS LOW FODMAP SO YOU CAN SUBSTITUTE THIS FOR THE NAPA CABBAGE IF YOU PREFER.

CHINESE PORK & VEGETABLES

PREPARATION TIME: 15 MINUTES
COOKING TIME: 20 MINUTES
SERVES: 4

Mix together the maple syrup, soy sauce, Chinese five-spice powder, Szechuan pepper, ginger, and 1 teaspoon of the sesame oil in a bowl. Add the pork to the bowl and massage the meat well with the mixture.

Heat a large, nonstick skillet over medium-high heat, then scrape the pork mixture into the pan and cook for 4 to 5 minutes, turning the pork slices over occasionally, until just cooked and tender.

Meanwhile, heat the remaining sesame oil in a wok over medium-high heat, then add the red pepper, Napa cabbage, bean sprouts, and baby bok choy. Stir-fry for 2 to 3 minutes, until just tender.

Remove the pork from the heat and serve immediately, scattered with the sesame seeds, with the stir-fried vegetables alongside.

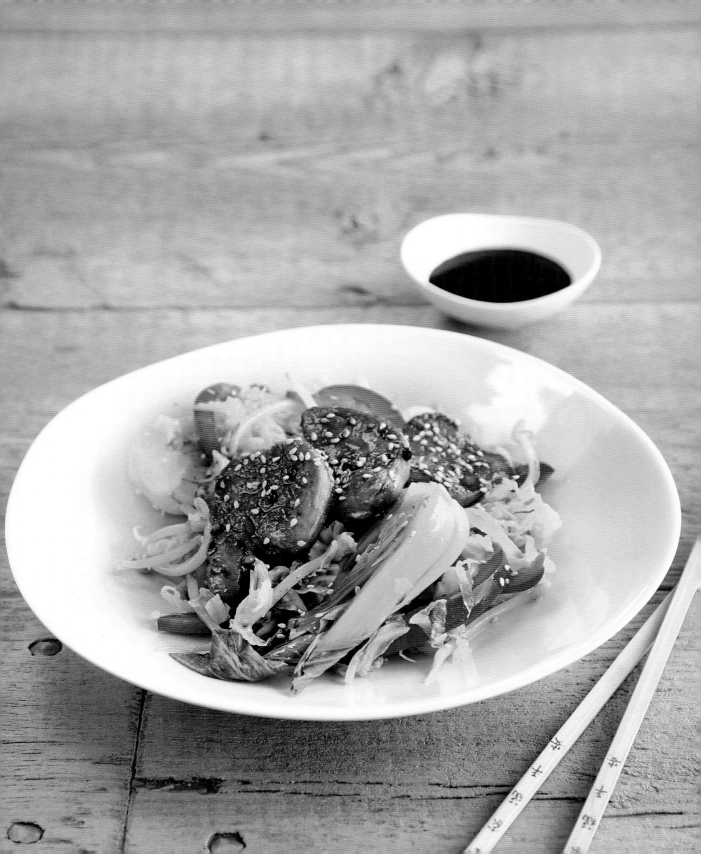

1 tablespoon garlic-infused oil

1 bunch of scallions (green parts only), sliced

1 to 2 hot green chiles, seeded and sliced

5 to 6 fresh curry leaves

1 tablespoon mild Low-FODMAP Curry Powder (*see page 47*)

¼ teaspoon turmeric

½ teaspoon fenugreek seeds

4 carrots, peeled and cut into thin matchsticks

9oz green snap beans, trimmed and halved

14fl oz can coconut milk

juice of 1 lime

salt and freshly ground black pepper

steamed rice or gluten-free bread, to serve (optional)

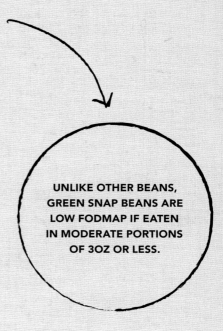

UNLIKE OTHER BEANS, GREEN SNAP BEANS ARE LOW FODMAP IF EATEN IN MODERATE PORTIONS OF 3OZ OR LESS.

SPICED CARROT & GREEN BEAN STEW

PREPARATION TIME: 10 MINUTES
COOKING TIME: 20 MINUTES
SERVES: 4

Heat the oil in a heavy saucepan. Add the scallions, chiles, and curry leaves and cook over medium heat for 1 to 2 minutes, until fragrant. Sprinkle with the curry powder, turmeric, and fenugreek seeds and season well.

Add the carrots and snap beans and cook, stirring, for a further 3 to 4 minutes, until everything is coated in the spices. Reduce the heat to low, pour in the coconut milk, and let simmer for 10 to 12 minutes or until the vegetables are tender.

Remove the saucepan from the heat and stir in the lime juice. Ladle the stew into warm bowls and serve with steamed rice or gluten-free bread, if liked.

butter or oil, for greasing

1lb 6oz potatoes, thinly sliced

1lb 2oz spinach

7oz mozzarella cheese, grated

4 vine tomatoes, sliced

3 eggs, beaten

$1\frac{1}{4}$ cups heavy whipping cream

salt and freshly ground black pepper

crisp salad, to serve

SPINACH & POTATO GRATIN

PREPARATION TIME: 10 MINUTES
COOKING TIME: 35 MINUTES
SERVES: 4

Preheat the oven to 350°F. Grease a large ovenproof dish.

Cook the potato slices in a large saucepan of salted boiling water for 5 minutes, then drain well.

Meanwhile, cook the spinach in a separate saucepan of boiling water for 1 to 2 minutes. Drain and squeeze out the excess water.

Arrange half the potato slices in a layer in the prepared ovenproof dish. Cover this layer with the spinach and half the mozzarella, seasoning each layer well with salt and pepper. Cover with the remaining potato slices and arrange the tomato slices on top. Scatter with the remaining mozzarella.

Beat the eggs and cream together in a bowl and season well with salt and pepper. Pour this mixture over the ingredients in the dish. Bake for about 30 minutes. Serve immediately with a salad.

¼ cup vegetable oil

1 bunch of scallions (green parts only), thinly sliced

1 red chile, slit lengthwise and seeded

1½-inch piece of fresh ginger root, peeled and shredded

2 plum tomatoes, finely diced

1 tablespoon Low-FODMAP Curry Powder (*see page 47*)

7fl oz canned coconut milk

1¾lb fresh clams, scrubbed

1 large handful of chopped cilantro leaves

3 tablespoons grated fresh coconut

TO SERVE (OPTIONAL)

salad

gluten-free crusty bread

SPICY CLAMS WITH COCONUT

PREPARATION TIME: 15 MINUTES
COOKING TIME: 20 MINUTES
SERVES: 4

Heat the oil in a large wok or saucepan over medium heat until hot. Add the scallions, red chile, and ginger and stir-fry for 3 to 4 minutes. Increase the heat to high, stir in the tomatoes, curry powder, and coconut milk and cook for a further 4 to 5 minutes.

Add the clams to the pan, discarding any that have cracked or don't shut when tapped on a hard surface, stir to mix, and cover the pan tightly with a lid. Continue to cook over high heat for 6 to 8 minutes, until the clams have opened. Discard any that remain closed.

Stir the chopped cilantro into the saucepan and scatter with the grated coconut. Ladle the mixture into bowls and serve immediately, with a fresh salad and crusty bread to mop up the juices, if liked.

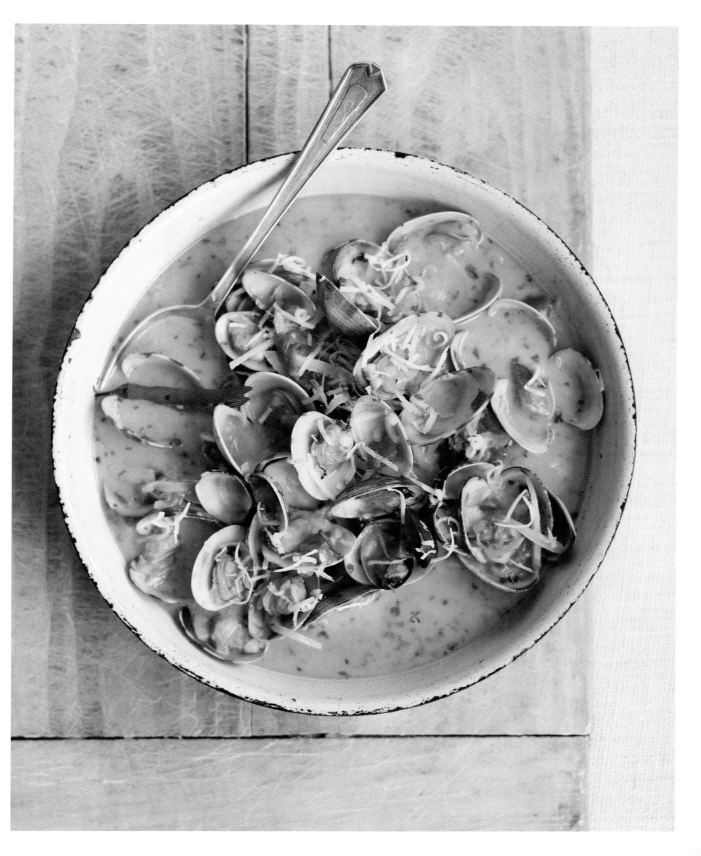

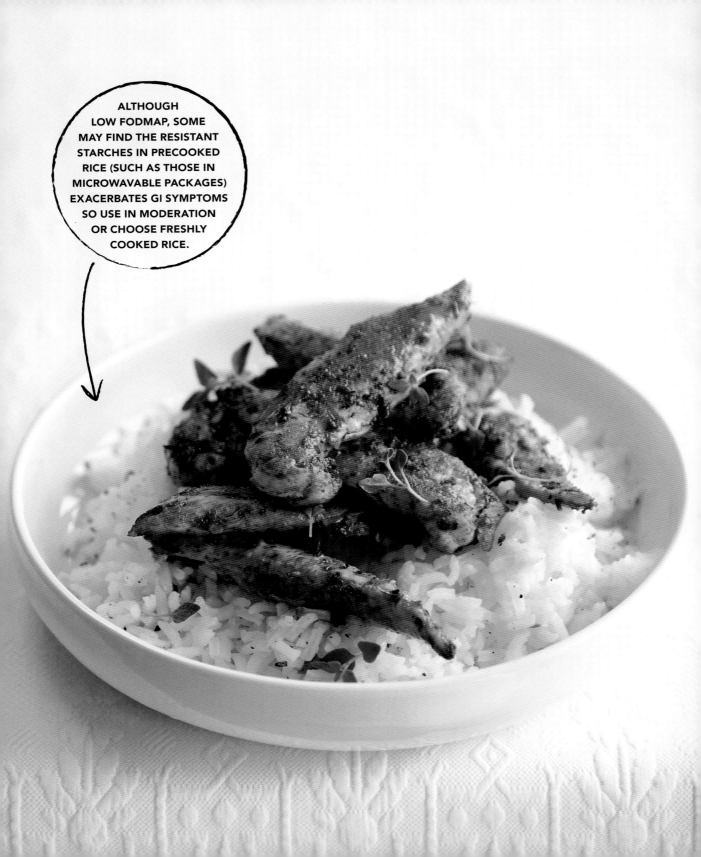

ALTHOUGH LOW FODMAP, SOME MAY FIND THE RESISTANT STARCHES IN PRECOOKED RICE (SUCH AS THOSE IN MICROWAVABLE PACKAGES) EXACERBATES GI SYMPTOMS SO USE IN MODERATION OR CHOOSE FRESHLY COOKED RICE.

- 2 tablespoons olive oil
- 1lb 2oz small chicken tenders
- sprigs of thyme, to garnish

FOR THE PIRI-PIRI SAUCE

- 1 teaspoon minced red chile
- 1 tablespoon garlic-infused olive oil
- ¼ teaspoon dried oregano
- ¼ teaspoon dried thyme
- 1 teaspoon paprika
- 2 tablespoons red wine vinegar

TO SERVE

- steamed rice
- crisp green salad (optional)

PIRI PIRI STIR-FRY

PREPARATION TIME: 5 MINUTES
COOKING TIME: 10 MINUTES
SERVES: 4

Heat the oil in a large, heavy wok or skillet over high heat. Add the chicken and cook, stirring occasionally, for 5 minutes, or until golden in places.

Mix all the piri-piri sauce ingredients together in a bowl and add the mixture to the pan with the chicken. Stir-fry for a further 3 to 4 minutes, stirring occasionally, until the chicken is cooked through and has absorbed the flavor of the sauce. Garnish with thyme sprigs.

Serve hot with steamed rice and a crisp green salad, if liked.

3 tablespoons light soy sauce

1 tablespoon peeled and finely grated fresh ginger root

1lb 2oz firm tofu, cut into 1/2-inch slices

2 tablespoons vegetable or peanut oil

1 carrot, peeled and cut into fine matchsticks

1lb 2oz bok choy, sliced

2 cups bean sprouts

8oz can bamboo shoots in water

1/4 cup oyster sauce

2 teaspoons golden sesame seeds, to garnish (optional)

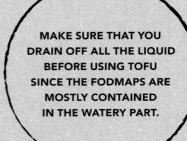

MAKE SURE THAT YOU DRAIN OFF ALL THE LIQUID BEFORE USING TOFU SINCE THE FODMAPS ARE MOSTLY CONTAINED IN THE WATERY PART.

MARINATED TOFU WITH VEGETABLES

PREPARATION TIME: 15 MINUTES, PLUS MARINATING
COOKING TIME: 15 MINUTES
SERVES: 4

Mix the soy sauce and ginger in a small bowl. Arrange the tofu slices in a shallow dish and pour in the soy and ginger marinade, gently turning the tofu over to coat. Set aside to marinate for about 20 minutes.

Preheat the broiler on the highest setting. Line a broiler pan with aluminum foil.

Carefully transfer the tofu slices to the foil-lined broiler pan, reserving the marinade. Cook under the hot broiler for about 3 minutes on each side, until golden. Remove from the heat and keep warm.

Meanwhile, heat the oil in a wok over medium heat. Add the carrot and bok choy and stir-fry for 4 to 5 minutes, until beginning to soften. Add the bean sprouts and bamboo shoots and cook for 1 minute, then pour in the remaining marinade and the oyster sauce.

Spoon the vegetables into deep bowls, top with the grilled tofu slices, and scatter with golden sesame seeds, if using. Serve immediately.

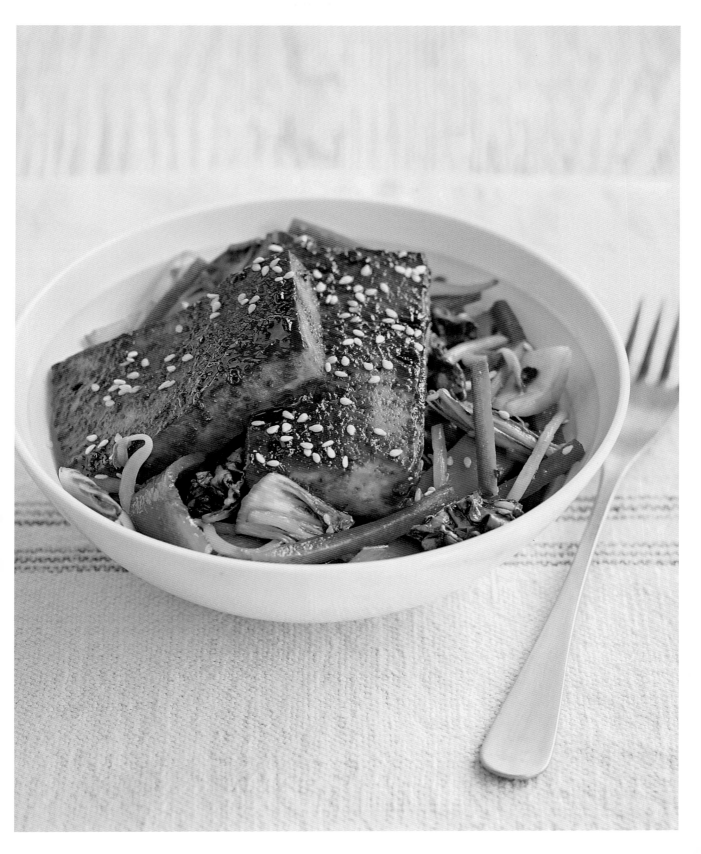

10$\frac{1}{2}$oz gluten-free penne

$\frac{1}{3}$ cup olive oil, divided

$\frac{3}{4}$ cup grated Parmesan cheese

handful of tarragon leaves

$\frac{1}{3}$ cup pine nuts, toasted

grated zest and juice of
1 lemon

3 tablespoons garlic-infused
olive oil

3 cooked chicken breasts,
sliced

3$\frac{1}{2}$oz watercress

12 baby tomatoes, quartered

CHICKEN & TARRAGON
PESTO PENNE

PREPARATION TIME: 20 MINUTES
COOKING TIME: 10 MINUTES
SERVES: 4

Cook the penne in a large saucepan of boiling water for 8 to 9 minutes or following the package directions. Drain and refresh under cold running water, then toss with 2 tablespoons of the olive oil.

Meanwhile, put the Parmesan, tarragon, pine nuts, and lemon zest into the bowl of a food processor and blend for 1 minute. Then, with the motor running, gradually pour in the remaining olive oil and the garlic-infused olive oil to form the pesto.

Transfer the pasta to a serving bowl. Add the chicken, watercress, tomatoes, lemon juice, and pesto and toss to mix. Serve immediately.

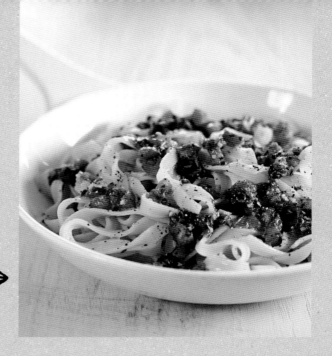

THE GARLIC-INFUSED OIL USED IN THIS RECIPE REPLACES THE ONION AND GARLIC THAT IS OFTEN USED IN TOMATO-BASED SAUCES, AND THE BASIL PROVIDES EXTRA DEPTH OF FLAVOR.

PASTA WITH TOMATO & BASIL SAUCE

PREPARATION TIME: 5 MINUTES
COOKING TIME: 10 MINUTES
SERVES: 4

14oz gluten-free spaghetti

3 tablespoons garlic-infused olive oil

2 tablespoons olive oil

6 ripe vine tomatoes, seeded and diced

1 cup loosely packed basil leaves

salt and freshly ground black pepper

Cook the pasta in a large saucepan of salted boiling water following the package directions.

Drain the pasta and return it to the pan. Add the oils, diced tomatoes, and basil leaves. Season to taste with salt and pepper and toss well to coat the pasta. Serve immediately.

13oz gluten-free fusilli pasta

⅓ cup pine nuts, toasted,
1 tablespoon reserved for
garnish

5½oz watercress, plus extra
sprigs to serve

⅓ cup extra-virgin olive oil

2 tablespoons garlic-infused
olive oil

5½oz crumbly low-lactose goat
cheese, plus extra to serve

salt and freshly ground
black pepper

SOME VARIETIES OF GOAT CHEESE ARE HIGHER IN LACTOSE THAN OTHERS. CHECK THE LABEL AND OPT FOR THOSE THAT CONTAIN LESS THAN 1 GRAM OF LACTOSE (LABELED AS SUGAR) PER 100 GRAMS OF CHEESE.

GOAT CHEESE & WATERCRESS PESTO PASTA

PREPARATION TIME: 10 MINUTES
COOKING TIME: 10 TO 12 MINUTES
SERVES: 4

Cook the pasta in a large saucepan of salted boiling water following the package directions, until al dente.

Meanwhile, put the pine nuts and watercress into the bowl of a food processor with a generous pinch of salt. Process for 15 seconds until coarsely chopped. Then, with the motor running, drizzle in the oils while you process for a further 20 seconds.

Drain the pasta thoroughly and tip it into a bowl. Crumble in the goat cheese and stir well. Season with pepper, then stir the pesto into the hot pasta. Divide the pasta between 4 serving plates and serve immediately with the reserved goat cheese, pine nuts, and some watercress sprigs.

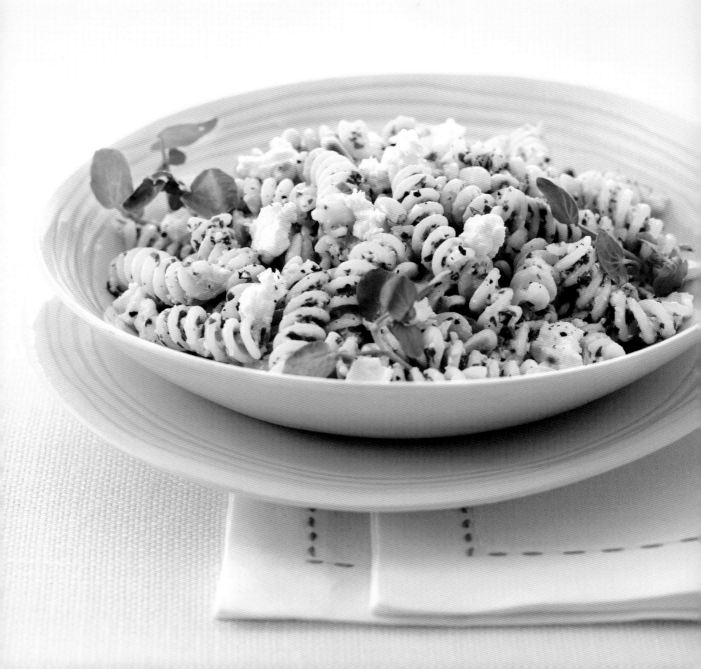

- 2 tablespoons garlic-infused olive oil
- 1 bunch of scallions (green parts only), chopped
- 14oz can cherry tomatoes
- ½ teaspoon dried red chile flakes
- pinch of sugar
- ½ teaspoon finely grated lemon zest
- 12oz gluten-free linguine or spaghetti
- 2 x 4¼oz cans sardines in oil, drained
- 2 teaspoons rinsed capers
- salt and freshly ground black pepper
- basil leaves, to garnish (optional)

SPICY SARDINE LINGUINE

PREPARATION TIME: 5 MINUTES
COOKING TIME: 20 MINUTES
SERVES: 4

Heat the olive oil in a large saucepan over medium heat. Add the scallions and cook for 1 minute, until softened. Add the tomatoes, chile flakes, sugar, and lemon zest and season with salt and pepper. Bring to a boil, then cover the pan with a lid and simmer for about 10 minutes, until thickened. Stir the sardines and capers into the tomato sauce for the final 1 to 2 minutes of the cooking time.

Meanwhile, cook the linguine in a large saucepan of boiling salted water following the package directions, until al dente. Drain, reserving 2 tablespoons of the cooking water, and return the pasta to the pan.

When the tomato sauce is ready, add it to the drained pasta along with the reserved cooking water and toss gently. Serve the mixture heaped in bowls, garnished with extra black pepper and with basil leaves, if desired.

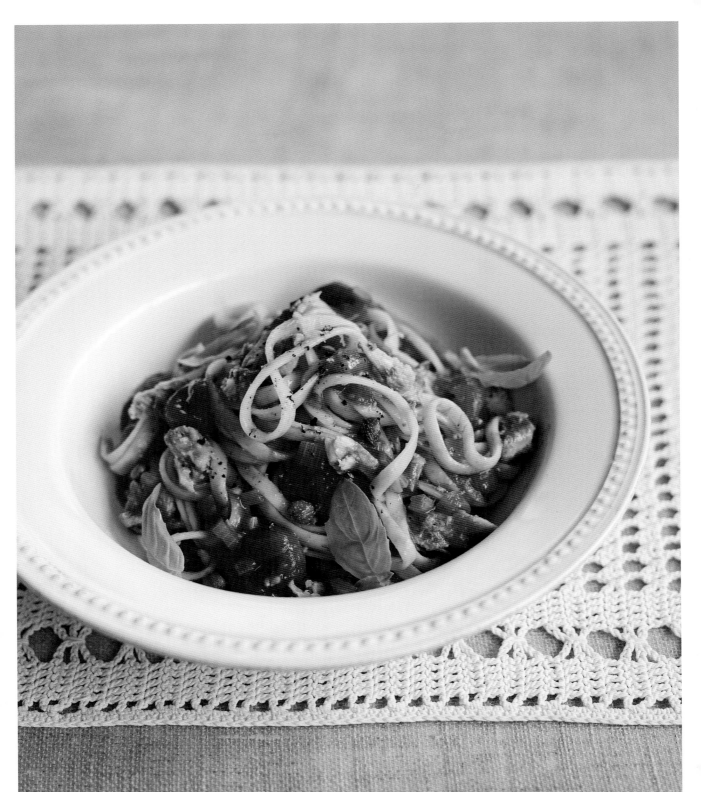

1¾lb russet potatoes, peeled and diced

1 egg yolk, beaten

1¼ cups gluten-free all-purpose flour

½ cup loosely packed basil leaves, finely shredded

½ cup grated Parmesan cheese

¼ cup extra-virgin olive oil

salt and freshly ground black pepper

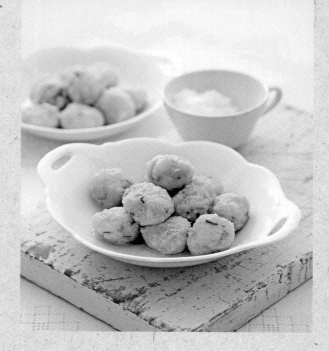

POTATO GNOCCHI

PREPARATION TIME: 20 MINUTES
COOKING TIME: 15 TO 20 MINUTES
SERVES: 4

Cook the potatoes in a saucepan of boiling water for 12 to 15 minutes, until soft. Drain and mash, or use a potato ricer to obtain a really smooth texture.

Place another saucepan of water on the heat to boil.

Transfer the mashed potatoes to a bowl and mix in the egg yolk, flour, and basil. Season with salt and pepper and stir well to combine.

Take 1 teaspoonful of the mixture into your hand and roll it into a walnut-sized ball. Press with the tines of a fork into a gnocchi shape. Set aside on a plate and repeat with the remaining mixture.

Drop the gnocchi into the saucepan of boiling water to cook—this should take only 1 to 2 minutes. The gnocchi will float when done.

Drain and toss the hot gnocchi in the grated Parmesan and olive oil and serve immediately.

CHERRY TOMATO & PEPPER TART

Grease a cookie sheet with vegetable oil and preheat the oven to 425°F.

Roll out the pastry thinly on a lightly floured surface and cut out a 10-inch circle. Transfer the dough circle to the prepared baking sheet. Using the tip of a sharp knife, score a continuous line around the circle ½ inch in from the edge of the pastry to form a border.

Mix the pesto in a bowl with the tomatoes, peppers, and feta. Spread the mixture in an even layer over the pastry, ensuring the filling is contained within the scored rim. Season with salt and pepper.

Place the cookie sheet on the upper rack of the oven and cook for 20 minutes, until the pastry is puffed up and golden (cover the tart with aluminum foil if the pastry starts to brown too quickly). Serve scattered with basil leaves to garnish.

PREPARATION TIME: 10 MINUTES
COOKING TIME: 25 MINUTES
SERVES: 4

vegetable oil, for greasing

13oz ready-made gluten-free puff pastry

gluten-free all-purpose flour, for dusting

¼ cup Low-FODMAP Pesto (see below)

1⅓ cups halved cherry tomatoes

5½oz mixed roasted bell peppers (if using ready-made, ensure the product is free from garlic), coarsely chopped

⅔ cup crumbled feta cheese

salt and freshly ground black pepper

basil leaves, to garnish

LOW-FODMAP PESTO

Ready-made pesto contains garlic and is off-limits when following a low-FODMAP diet. The recipe below produces a tasty homemade alternative.

Put 1 cup firmly packed basil leaves, 3 tablespoons of pine nuts, 1 tablespoon of garlic-infused olive oil, ¼ cup extra-virgin olive oil, and some salt and pepper into the bowl of a food processor and process until fairly smooth. Transfer to a bowl, stir in 2 tablespoons of freshly grated Parmesan cheese, and adjust the seasoning to taste.

4 chicken breasts,
about $\frac{1}{4}$lb each
....

$\frac{1}{2}$ cup firmly packed
basil leaves
....

2 tablespoons garlic-infused
olive oil
....

2 tablespoons pine nuts,
toasted
....

2 tablespoons grated
Parmesan cheese
....

$\frac{2}{3}$ cup tightly packed arugula
....

$3\frac{1}{2}$ cups boiling water
....

$1\frac{1}{3}$ cups polenta
....

salt and freshly ground
black pepper

CHICKEN
WITH PESTO & POLENTA

PREPARATION TIME: 15 MINUTES
COOKING TIME: 10 MINUTES
SERVES: 4

Preheat the broiler on the highest setting.

Slice each chicken breast in half horizontally through the middle and season all 8 pieces. Arrange the pieces in a broiler pan.

Put the basil, oil, pine nuts, Parmesan, and arugula into the bowl of a food processor or blender and process until finely chopped. Set aside.

Cook the chicken under the hot broiler for 5 to 7 minutes, until just cooked through and still succulent.

Meanwhile, lightly salt the measured boiling water in a saucepan and stir in the polenta. Cook over medium heat, stirring constantly, for about 2 minutes, until thickened. Stir the arugula pesto through the polenta.

Serve the chicken slices on top of the polenta.

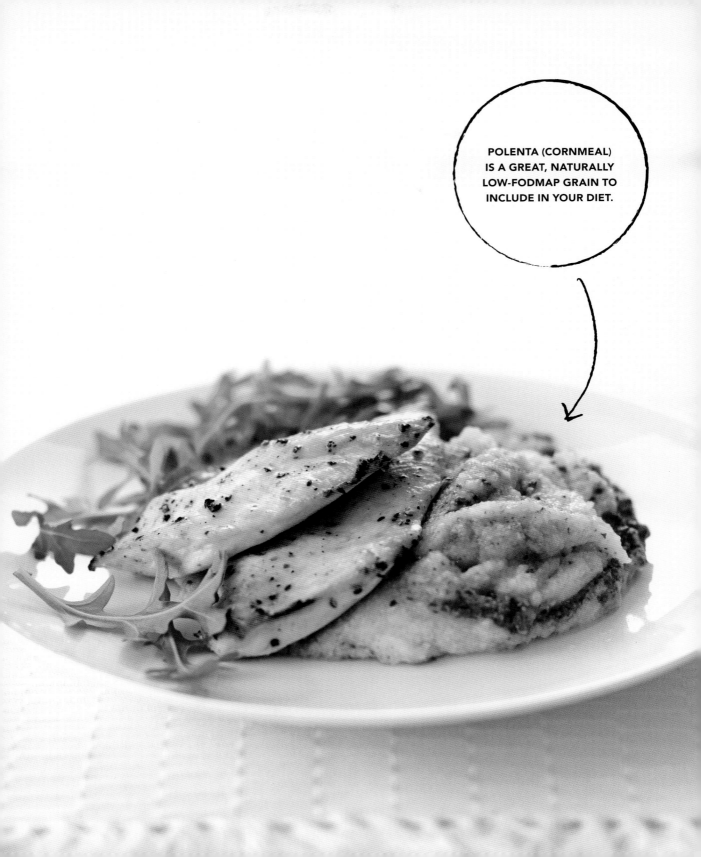

POLENTA (CORNMEAL) IS A GREAT, NATURALLY LOW-FODMAP GRAIN TO INCLUDE IN YOUR DIET.

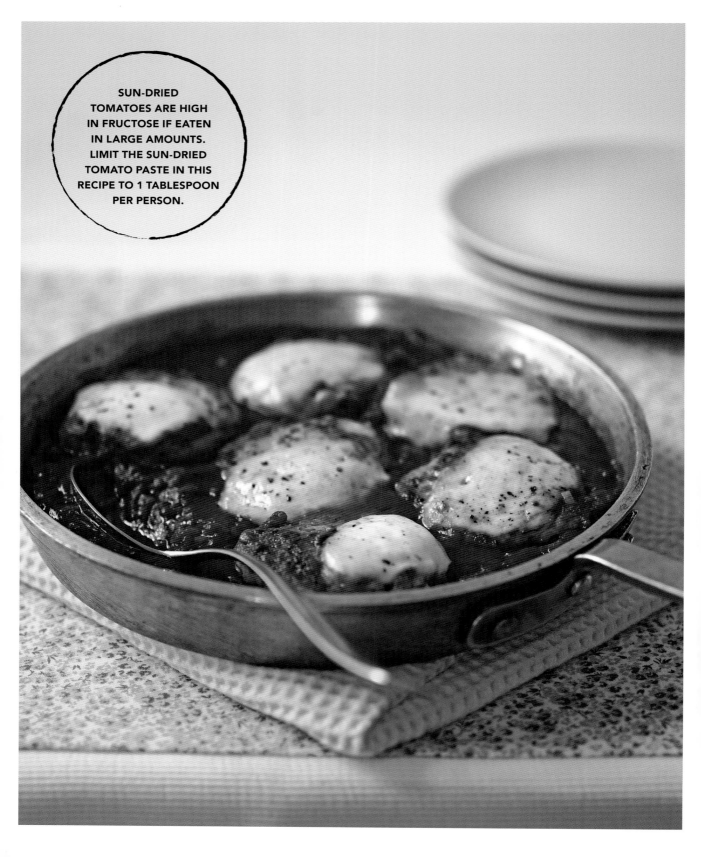

SUN-DRIED
TOMATOES ARE HIGH
IN FRUCTOSE IF EATEN
IN LARGE AMOUNTS.
LIMIT THE SUN-DRIED
TOMATO PASTE IN THIS
RECIPE TO 1 TABLESPOON
PER PERSON.

- 1lb 2oz ground turkey
- handful of fresh chives, snipped
- 1¾oz can anchovies, drained and chopped
- ⅔ cup fresh gluten-free bread crumbs
- ¼ cup olive oil, divided
- 2 x 14oz cans diced tomatoes
- 2 tablespoons sun-dried tomato paste
- 2 teaspoons dried oregano
- 1 bunch of scallions (green parts only), sliced
- 1 tablespoon light brown sugar
- 4oz mozzarella cheese, thinly sliced
- salt and freshly ground black pepper
- warmed gluten-free crusty bread, to serve (optional)

TURKEY POLPETTES
WITH TOMATOES

PREPARATION TIME: 15 MINUTES
COOKING TIME: 30 MINUTES
SERVES: 4

Mix together the turkey, chives, anchovies, bread crumbs, and a little salt and pepper in a bowl. Divide the mixture into 8 portions and shape each of these into a flat patty.

Heat 2 tablespoons of the oil in a large ovenproof skillet over medium heat. Add the patties and fry for 8 minutes, until golden on both sides. Transfer to a plate.

Add the remaining oil to the same skillet. Stir in the tomatoes, tomato paste, oregano, scallions, sugar, and a little salt and pepper and bring to a simmer.

Return the patties to the pan, pushing them down into the sauce. Cook gently, uncovered, for 15 minutes, until the patties are cooked through.

Meanwhile, preheat the broiler on a medium setting.

Place the mozzarella slices on top of the mixture in the skillet and season with plenty of pepper. Transfer the pan to the broiler and let broil until the cheese melts. Serve with warmed gluten-free crusty bread, if liked.

3 tablespoons chopped fresh mixed herbs (such as chives, parsley, rosemary, and oregano), divided

1 tablespoon garlic-infused olive oil, divided

finely grated zest of 1 lemon

4 thick fillets of white fish (such as cod, haddock, or pollock), about 5½oz each

2¼lb russet potatoes, peeled and cut into chunks

2 tablespoons lemon juice

½ cup grated Parmesan cheese

¼ cup olive oil

salt and freshly ground black pepper

steamed green snap beans, to serve (limit each portion to 3oz)

GRIDDLED FISH WITH LEMON
WITH MASHED POTATOES & PARMESAN

PREPARATION TIME: 20 MINUTES
COOKING TIME: 30 MINUTES
SERVES: 4

Mix 1 tablespoon of the chopped herbs with a little of the garlic-infused oil, lemon zest, and some seasoning, then massage the mixture into the fish fillets. Marinate for 10 to 15 minutes.

Meanwhile, cook the potatoes in a large saucepan of lightly salted boiling water for 12 to 15 minutes, or until tender.

Heat a griddle until hot. Add the fish, skin-side down, and cook for 4 to 5 minutes, until the skin is crisp. Turn the fish over, turn off the heat, and set aside for 3 to 4 minutes, until cooked. Keep the fish warm.

Drain the potatoes, then return them to the pan over very low heat. Let steam for 1 to 2 minutes to dry out the potatoes. Add the lemon juice, Parmesan cheese, remaining herbs, the remaining garlic-infused oil, and the olive oil. Season to taste and mash until smooth, then spoon onto 4 warmed plates. Serve the mashed potatoes with the griddled fish and some steamed green snap beans.

1½lb round white potatoes, thinly sliced

⅓ cup olive oil, divided

1 tablespoon chopped thyme

4 sea bream fillets, about 5½oz each

2¾oz prosciutto, chopped

1 bunch of scallions (green parts only), finely chopped

finely grated zest of 1 lemon

7oz samphire

salt and freshly ground black pepper

STUFFED BREAM WITH SAMPHIRE

PREPARATION TIME: 20 MINUTES
COOKING TIME: 55 MINUTES
SERVES: 4

Preheat the oven to 375°F.

In a large bowl, toss the potato slices with ¼ cup of the oil, a little salt and pepper, and the thyme. Tip the mixture into a roasting pan or ovenproof dish and spread it out in an even layer. Cover the pan or dish with aluminum foil and bake for about 30 minutes, until the potatoes are tender.

Score the bream fillets several times with a sharp knife.

Mix the prosciutto with the scallions, lemon zest, and a little black pepper in a bowl. Use this mixture to sandwich the bream fillets together in pairs. Tie each bundle at intervals with kitchen string. Cut each bundle of sandwiched fillets through the center to make 4 evenly sized portions.

Lay the fish over the potatoes in the baking pan and return the pan to the oven, uncovered, for a further 20 minutes or until the fish is cooked through.

Scatter the samphire around the fish and drizzle with the remaining oil. Return the pan to the oven for a further 5 minutes, then serve.

2 tablespoons garlic-infused olive oil

1 bunch of scallions (green parts only), sliced

1 tablespoon tomato paste

14oz can diced tomatoes

pinch of sugar

handful of thyme leaves

4 skinless cod fillets, about $\frac{1}{4}$lb each

$\frac{1}{4}$ cup pitted black olives

salt and freshly ground black pepper

TO SERVE (OPTIONAL)

new potatoes

low-FODMAP vegetables

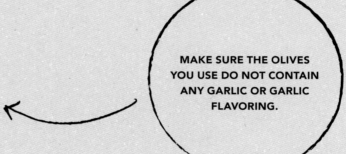

MAKE SURE THE OLIVES YOU USE DO NOT CONTAIN ANY GARLIC OR GARLIC FLAVORING.

COD IN TOMATO & OLIVE SAUCE

PREPARATION TIME: 5 MINUTES
COOKING TIME: 20 TO 25 MINUTES
SERVES: 4

Heat the oil in a large, deep skillet over medium heat. Add the scallions and tomato paste and cook for 1 minute, then pour in the tomatoes. Add the sugar and thyme. Season, reduce the heat, and let simmer for 10 minutes.

Slide the fish fillets into the sauce along with the olives, cover loosely with aluminum foil, and simmer for 8 to 10 minutes, or until the fish flakes easily. Serve with some boiled new potatoes and your choice of low-FODMAP vegetables, if liked.

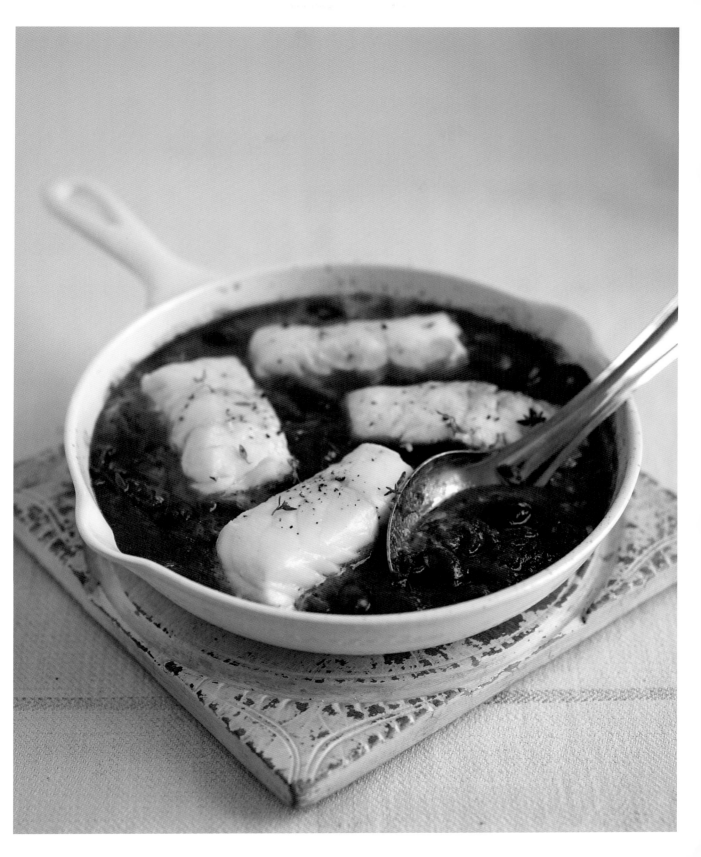

- 1¼ cups brown rice
- 1 eggplant, cut into chunks
- 3 zucchini, cut into chunks
- ¼ cup flat-leaf parsley, chopped, plus extra to serve
- 1 tablespoon rosemary, chopped
- ⅔ cup olive oil
- grated zest and juice of 2 lemons
- 9oz cherry tomatoes
- ⅔ cup blanched peanuts
- 2 carrots, peeled and grated
- 2 tablespoons light soy sauce
- freshly ground black pepper

LIMIT PEANUTS TO A SMALL HANDFUL PER PORTION TO ENSURE THIS DISH REMAINS LOW FODMAP.

LEMON-DRESSED MIXED VEGETABLE KEBABS
WITH NUT PILAF

PREPARATION TIME: 20 MINUTES
COOKING TIME: 15 MINUTES
SERVES: 4

Cook the rice following the package directions. Drain and refresh under cold running water, then drain again.

Meanwhile, preheat the broiler on the highest setting. Soak 8 wooden skewers in water.

Place the eggplant and zucchini in a large bowl. Put the parsley and rosemary into a pitcher with the olive oil and the lemon zest and juice and whisk together. Season with pepper, then pour the mixture over the vegetables and toss together.

Thread the dressed vegetables with the tomatoes onto the wooden skewers. Cook the skewers under the hot broiler (alternatively, cook them on a barbecue), turning occasionally, for 8 to 10 minutes, until lightly charred and tender.

Toss the cooled rice with the peanuts, carrots, the remaining parsley, and the soy sauce. Season with a little pepper. Serve the hot kebabs on a bed of the rice salad.

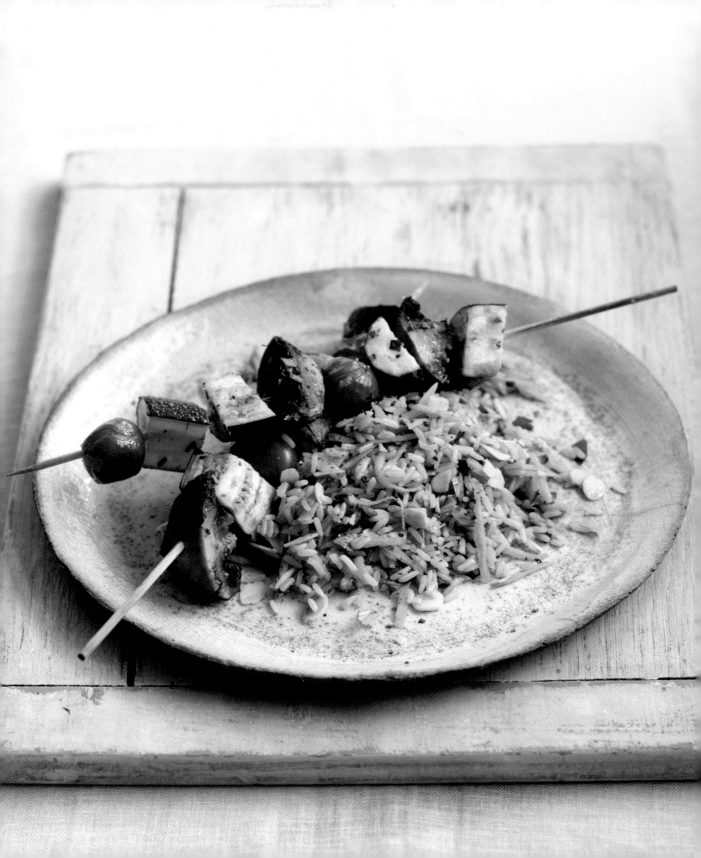

CHECK THAT YOUR ENGLISH MUSTARD IS FREE FROM ONION AND GARLIC TO ENSURE THIS RECIPE REMAINS LOW FODMAP.

SALMON WITH LIME ZUCCHINI

PREPARATION TIME: 15 MINUTES
COOKING TIME: 15 TO 20 MINUTES
SERVES: 4

4 salmon fillets, about 5½oz each
....
1 tablespoon English mustard
....
2 teaspoons peeled and grated fresh ginger root
....
2 teaspoons maple syrup
....
1 tablespoon light soy sauce
....

FOR THE LIME ZUCCHINI

1lb 2oz zucchini, thinly sliced lengthwise
....
2 tablespoons olive oil
....
grated zest and juice of 1 lime
....
2 tablespoons chopped mint
....
salt and freshly ground black pepper

Preheat the broiler on the highest setting.

Place the salmon fillets, skin-side down, in a shallow ovenproof dish, ensuring they fit in the dish snugly in a single layer.

Mix the mustard, ginger, maple syrup, and soy sauce in a bowl, then spoon this mixture evenly over the salmon.

Make the lime zucchini. Heat a ridged grill pan. Put the zucchini and oil into a plastic bag, seal, and shake well. Then remove the zucchini slices from the bag and cook them on the ridged grill pan over medium heat for about 5 minutes, until lightly charred on each side and tender. You may need to do this in batches.

Stir the lime zest and juice, mint, and seasoning together in a bowl.

While the zucchini are cooking, broil the salmon fillets for 10 to 15 minutes, depending on thickness, until lightly charred on top and cooked through.

Transfer the salmon to serving plates. Arrange the zucchini slices around the fish and drizzle them with lime dressing. Serve hot.

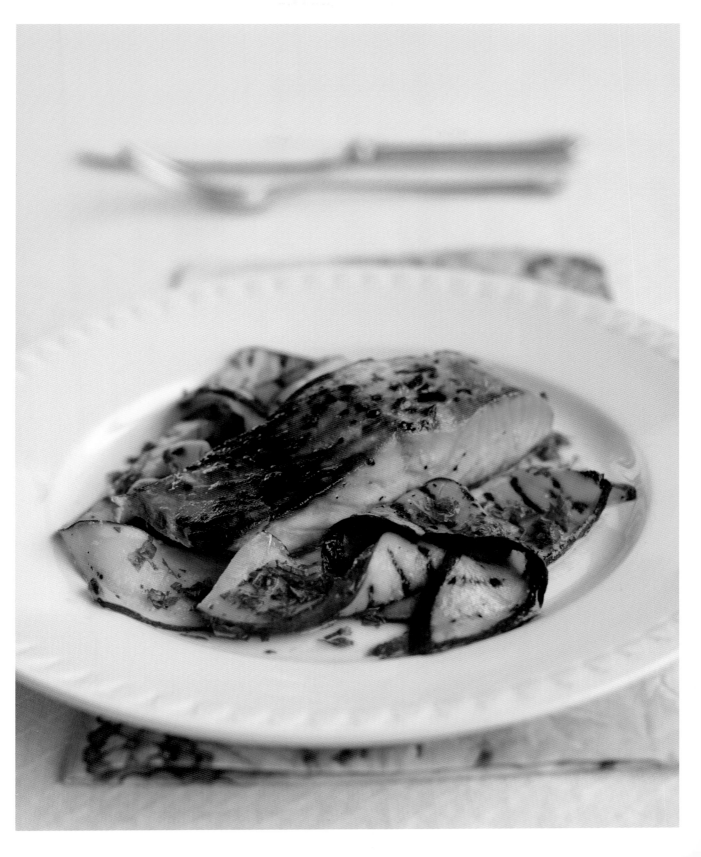

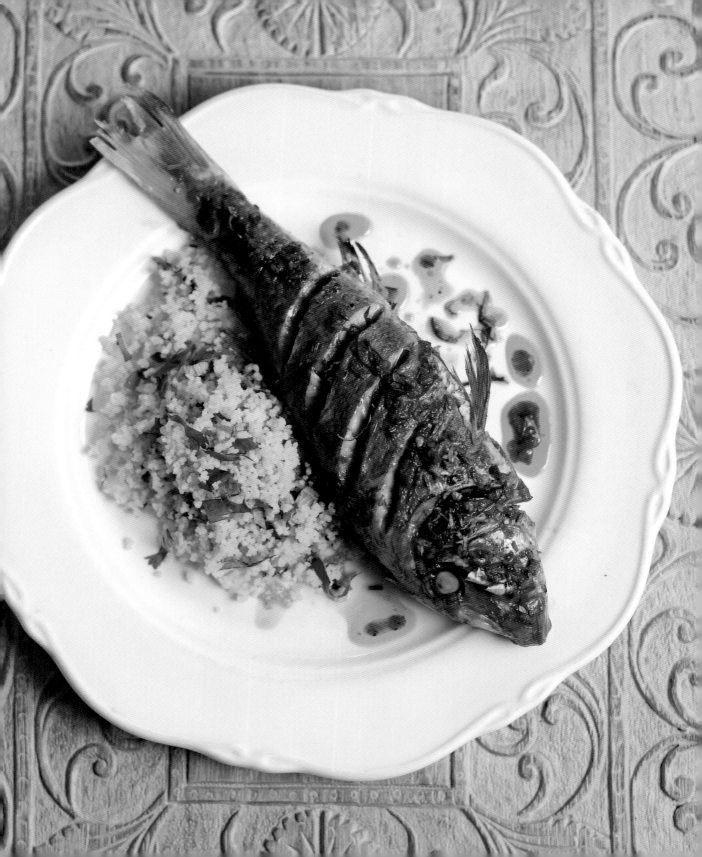

oil, for greasing

4 whole red mullet, about
¼lb each

small bunch of flat-leaf
parsley, coarsely chopped,
to garnish

gluten-free couscous,
to serve

FOR THE CHERMOULA SAUCE

1 teaspoon saffron threads

2 teaspoons water

1 red chile, seeded
and chopped

1 to 2 teaspoons cumin seeds

1 teaspoon sea salt

¼ cup garlic-infused
olive oil

¼ cup lemon juice

small bunch of fresh cilantro,
finely chopped

handful of chives, snipped

freshly ground black pepper

BROILED RED MULLET
WITH CHERMOULA SAUCE

PREPARATION TIME: 15 MINUTES,
   PLUS SOAKING
COOKING TIME: 10 MINUTES
SERVES: 4

Preheat the broiler on the highest setting. Oil a broiler pan.

Make the sauce first. Place the saffron in a small bowl with the measured water and let soak for 5 minutes.

Using a mortar and pestle, pound the chile, cumin seeds, and salt to form a coarse paste, then gradually beat in the oil and lemon juice. Then stir in the cilantro and chives and season with pepper. Add the saffron water and mix well.

Make 3 to 4 slashes on both sides of each fish. Place the fish on the prepared broiler pan and brush with a little of the sauce. Cook under the hot broiler for 4 to 5 minutes, then turn the fish over and brush with a little more sauce. Broil for 3 to 4 minutes, until cooked through.

Meanwhile, heat the remaining sauce in a small saucepan. Place each fish on a serving dish, drizzle each one with the sauce, and garnish with the parsley. Serve with couscous.

SIDE DISHES

½ stick butter

2¼lb whole baby carrots,
or young carrots, quartered
lengthwise

generous pinch of sugar

juice of 1 orange

salt and freshly ground
black pepper

flat-leaf parsley, coarsely
chopped, to garnish

GLAZED BABY CARROTS

PREPARATION TIME: 5 MINUTES
COOKING TIME: 15 TO 20 MINUTES
SERVES: 6

Melt the butter in a saucepan. Add the carrots and sugar and season with salt and pepper. Pour in just enough water to cover the carrots and cook over very low heat, uncovered, for 10 to 12 minutes or until the carrots are tender and the liquid has evaporated. As the water evaporates, add the orange juice.

Serve garnished with chopped parsley.

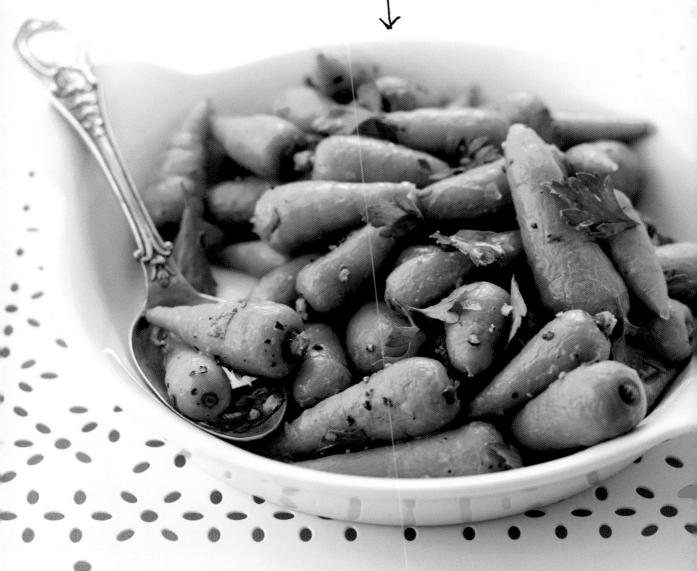

A DELICIOUS LOW-FODMAP ALTERNATIVE TO THE POPULAR HONEY-GLAZED CARROTS, AND JUST AS SWEET AND DELICIOUS.

4 baking potatoes,
6 to 9oz each, peeled
and halved lengthwise

....

¼ cup olive oil

....

2 tablespoons sesame seeds

....

salt

POTATOES ROASTED
WITH SESAME SEEDS

PREPARATION TIME: 10 MINUTES
COOKING TIME: 1 TO 1¼ HOURS
SERVES: 4

Preheat the oven to 400°F.

Place the potatoes on your cutting board with the cut sides facing down. Using a sharp knife, make cuts at ¼-inch intervals along the length of each piece of potato, almost through to the base, so that they just hold together.

Heat the oil in a roasting pan in the oven until hot. Add the potatoes to the pan and drizzle the hot oil evenly over them. Then sprinkle with a little salt, baste well, and roast for 30 minutes.

After the cooking time has elapsed, remove the potatoes from the oven and sprinkle with the sesame seeds. Return the pan to the oven and bake for a further 30 minutes or until the potatoes are golden brown and crisp.

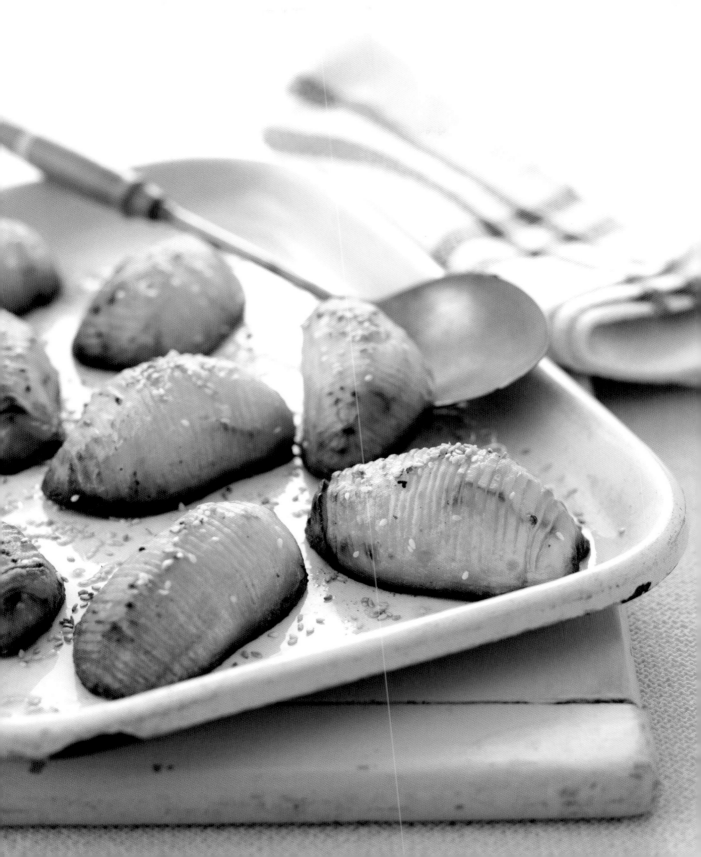

3 tablespoons ghee or butter

¼ cup finely chopped fresh
cilantro, plus extra
to garnish

rind of 1 preserved lemon,
finely sliced

2¼lb potatoes,
peeled and finely sliced

salt and freshly ground
black pepper

POTATOES ROASTED WITH CILANTRO & PRESERVED LEMON

PREPARATION TIME: 10 MINUTES
COOKING TIME: 25 MINUTES
SERVES: 4

Preheat the oven to 400°F.

Melt the ghee or butter in a small saucepan and stir in the cilantro and preserved lemon rind.

Put the potatoes into a large bowl, pour the melted mixture over them, and toss well to coat.

Spread the coated potatoes in an ovenproof dish, season, and cover the dish with aluminum foil. Bake for 15 minutes, then remove the foil and return the dish to the oven for a further 10 minutes, until the potatoes are tender and lightly browned.

Garnish with the extra cilantro and serve alongside roasted or broiled meat, poultry, or fish.

1lb 6oz baby parsnips, scrubbed

1 tablespoon garlic-infused olive oil

2 sprigs of thyme, leaves picked and chopped

1 teaspoon grated lemon zest

pinch of cayenne pepper

pinch of sea salt

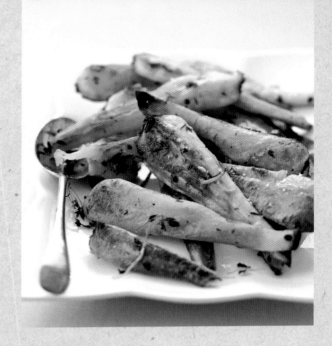

ROAST PARSNIPS WITH THYME BUTTER

PREPARATION TIME: 10 MINUTES
COOKING TIME: 40 TO 45 MINUTES
SERVES: 4

Preheat the oven to 400°F.

Put all the ingredients into a large bowl and toss to coat the parsnips in the seasoned oil. Transfer to a roasting pan. Bake for 40 to 45 minutes, stirring occasionally, until golden and tender. Serve immediately.

½ cup olive oil

1 bunch of scallions (green parts only), sliced

1 eggplant, cut into bite-sized cubes

2 large zucchini, cut into bite-sized pieces

1 red bell pepper, seeded and cut into bite-sized pieces

1 yellow bell pepper, seeded and cut into bite-sized pieces

14oz can diced tomatoes

¼ cup chopped flat-leaf parsley or basil

salt and freshly ground black pepper

PACKED FULL OF VEGETABLES, THIS DISH IS GOOD FOR COMBATING CONSTIPATION BY PROVIDING VITAL SOLUBLE FIBER.

QUICK ONE-POT RATATOUILLE

PREPARATION TIME: 10 MINUTES
COOKING TIME: 20 MINUTES
SERVES: 4

Heat the oil in a large saucepan over medium heat until very hot. Add the scallions, eggplant, zucchini, and peppers and cook, stirring constantly, for a few minutes, until the vegetables have softened. Add the tomatoes, season to taste with salt and pepper, and stir well.

Reduce the heat, cover the pan tightly with a lid, and let simmer for 15 minutes, until all the vegetables are cooked. Remove from the heat and stir in the chopped parsley or basil before serving.

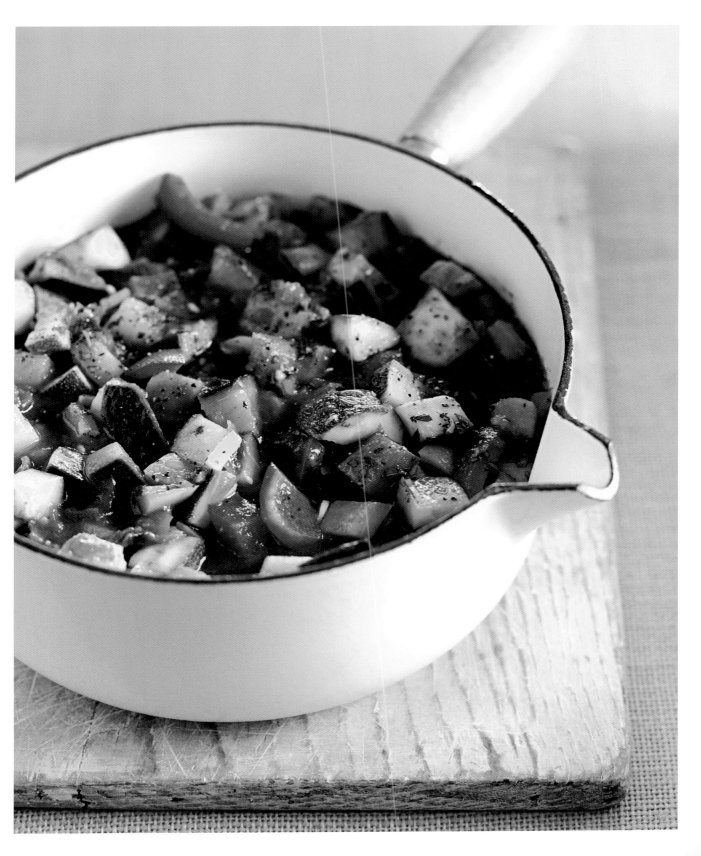

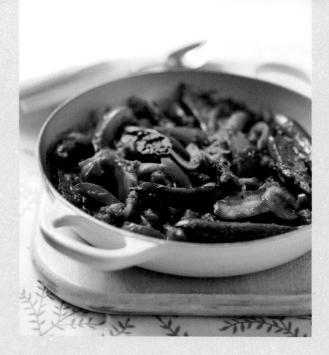

- ⅓ cup garlic-infused olive oil, divided
- 1 bunch of scallions (green parts only), sliced
- 7oz can diced tomatoes
- 1 green bell pepper, seeded and sliced
- 1 eggplant or 3 baby eggplants, sliced
- 1 large zucchini or 4 baby zucchini, sliced
- salt and freshly ground black pepper

BRAISED SPANISH VEGETABLES

PREPARATION TIME: 10 MINUTES
COOKING TIME: 35 MINUTES
SERVES: 4 TO 6

Heat 1 tablespoon of the oil in a large skillet over medium heat. Add the scallions and cook for 5 to 7 minutes, until softened. Add the tomatoes and a splash of water and let simmer for 15 minutes.

Meanwhile, heat 1 tablespoon of the oil in a separate skillet. Add the green pepper and cook for 5 minutes, stirring, until softened and lightly browned. Remove the pepper from the pan and set aside. Pour another 2 tablespoons of the oil into the pan. Add the eggplant and cook for 5 minutes, until golden, then set aside. Add the remaining oil to the pan, add the zucchini and cook for 5 minutes, until golden.

Return the pepper and eggplant to the pan, pour in the tomato sauce, and season well. Bring to a boil, then reduce the heat and simmer for 10 minutes, until the vegetables are very tender and most of the liquid has evaporated.

4 zucchini
....
1 cup diced plum tomatoes
....
1½ cups mozzarella cheese,
grated
....
2 tablespoons shredded
basil leaves
....
¼ cup grated Parmesan cheese
....
salt and freshly ground
black pepper

STUFFED ZUCCHINI

PREPARATION TIME: 15 MINUTES
COOKING TIME: 30 MINUTES
SERVES: 4

Preheat the oven to 400°F.

Slice the zucchini in half horizontally, then scoop out the center of each half, reserving the flesh. Place the zucchini halves in a roasting pan and bake for 10 minutes, until slightly softened.

Meanwhile, chop the reserved zucchini flesh and mix it in a bowl with the chopped tomatoes, grated mozzarella, and basil. Season with salt and pepper.

Remove the zucchini halves from the oven and spoon the filling into each zucchini shell. Sprinkle the filling with the grated Parmesan and return the pan to the oven. Bake for a further 15 minutes, until golden.

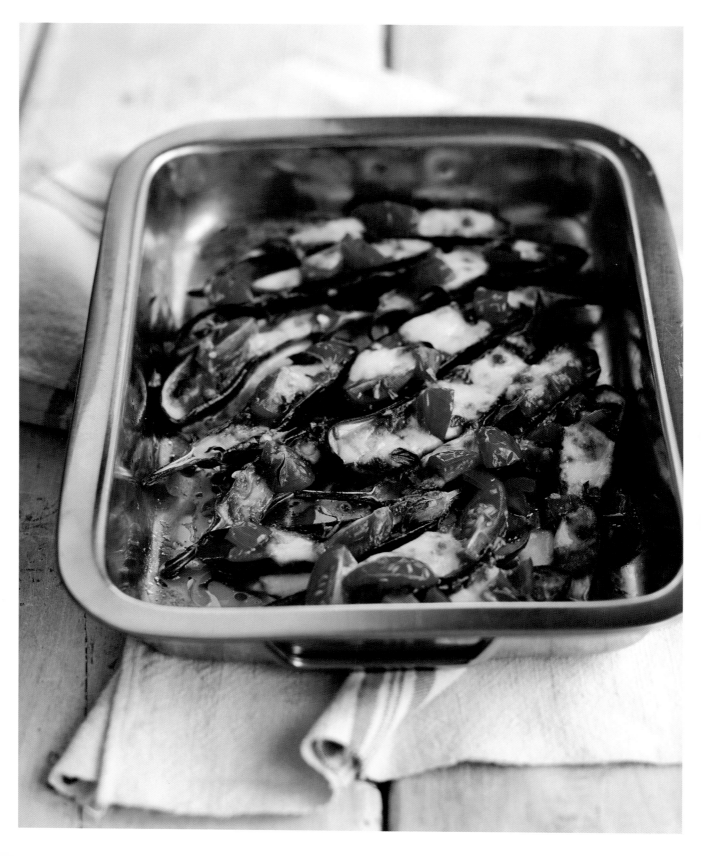

⅓ cup olive oil

12 baby eggplants, halved

½ cup tomato purée (free from sun-dried tomatoes)

½ cup chopped tomatoes

pinch of dried red chili flakes

handful of oregano leaves, chopped

7oz mozzarella cheese, sliced

salt and freshly ground black pepper

THE AMOUNT OF LACTOSE IN MOZZARELLA CAN VARY, SO WHILE IN THE ELIMINATION STAGES OF THE LOW-FODMAP DIET LIMIT MOZZARELLA TO 1¾OZ PER PORTION.

EGGPLANT, TOMATO & MOZZARELLA MELTS

PREPARATION TIME: 10 MINUTES
COOKING TIME: 20 MINUTES
SERVES: 4

Preheat the broiler on the highest setting.

Rub the oil over the eggplants and season well. Place them on a broiler pan and cook under the hot broiler for 5 to 7 minutes on each side or until soft and golden brown.

Mix together the tomato purée, fresh tomatoes, chili flakes, and oregano and season well. Arrange the eggplants on the broiler pan with their cut sides facing up. Spoon a little of the purée mixture onto each eggplant half and place some mozzarella slices on top. Broil for 2 to 3 minutes, until the mozzarella has just melted and serve immediately.

4 red or yellow bell peppers, halved and seeded

4 small tomatoes, halved

7oz feta cheese, sliced

3 scallions (green parts only), thinly sliced

2 tablespoons olive oil or vegetable oil, plus extra for greasing

1⅓ cups gluten-free couscous

2 tablespoons butter

freshly ground black pepper

2 tablespoons pumpkin or sunflower seeds, to garnish (optional)

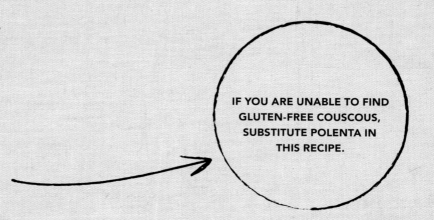

IF YOU ARE UNABLE TO FIND GLUTEN-FREE COUSCOUS, SUBSTITUTE POLENTA IN THIS RECIPE.

BAKED PEPPERS
WITH FETA & SCALLIONS

PREPARATION TIME: 10 MINUTES
COOKING TIME: 25 MINUTES
SERVES: 4

Preheat the oven to 400°F. Lightly grease a baking pan.

Put the pepper halves, cut-side up, onto the prepared baking pan. Fill the recesses with the tomato halves, feta slices, and scallions. Season with black pepper and drizzle with the oil. Bake for 20 to 25 minutes, until softened and golden.

Meanwhile, put the couscous into a bowl with the butter and add 1¼ cups boiling water. Cover the bowl and set aside for 5 to 8 minutes, until the liquid has been absorbed and the grains are tender.

Serve the baked peppers with the couscous, scattered with pumpkin or sunflower seeds, if using.

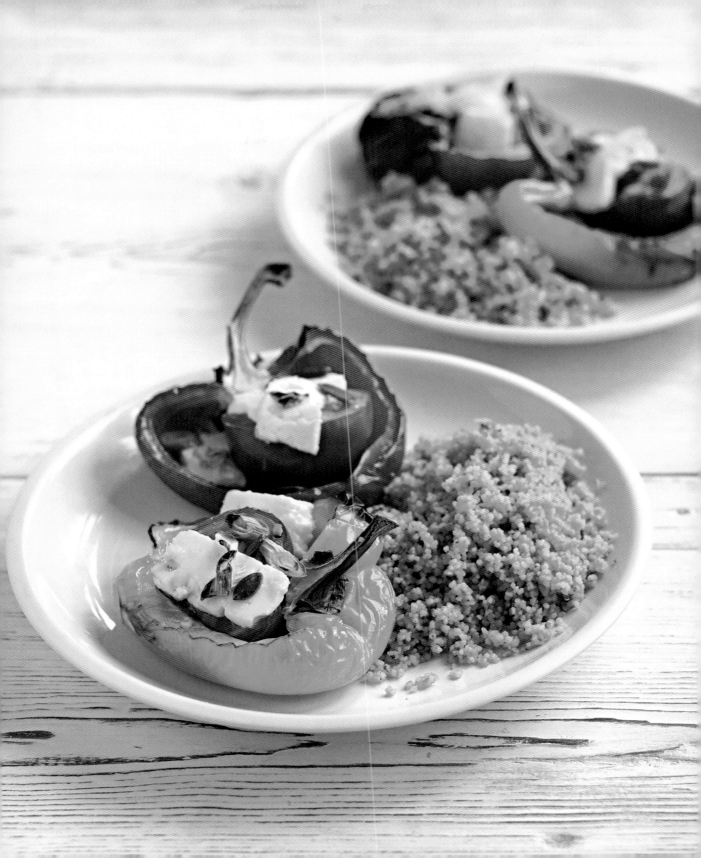

spray oil, for oiling

1 quart water

2 teaspoons salt

1¼ cups polenta

½ stick butter

½ cup grated Parmesan cheese,
plus extra to serve

olive oil, for brushing

freshly ground black pepper

chopped flat-leaf parsley,
to garnish

CHARGRILLED POLENTA TRIANGLES

PREPARATION TIME: 10 MINUTES,
PLUS COOLING
COOKING TIME: 15 TO 20 MINUTES
SERVES: 8

Lightly oil a 9 x 12 inch baking pan with spray oil.

Bring the measured water to a boil in a heavy saucepan. Add the salt, then gradually whisk in the polenta in a steady stream. Cook over low heat, stirring constantly with a wooden spoon, for 5 minutes, until the grains have swelled and thickened.

Remove the pan from the heat and immediately beat in the butter, Parmesan, and pepper until smooth. Pour the mixture into the prepared pan and let cool.

Turn out the polenta onto a cutting board and slice it into large squares. Cut each square diagonally in half into triangles. Brush the triangles with a little oil.

Heat a griddle until hot over medium-high heat. Add the polenta triangles, in batches, and cook for 2 to 3 minutes on each side, until charred and heated through. Serve immediately, garnished with grated Parmesan and chopped parsley.

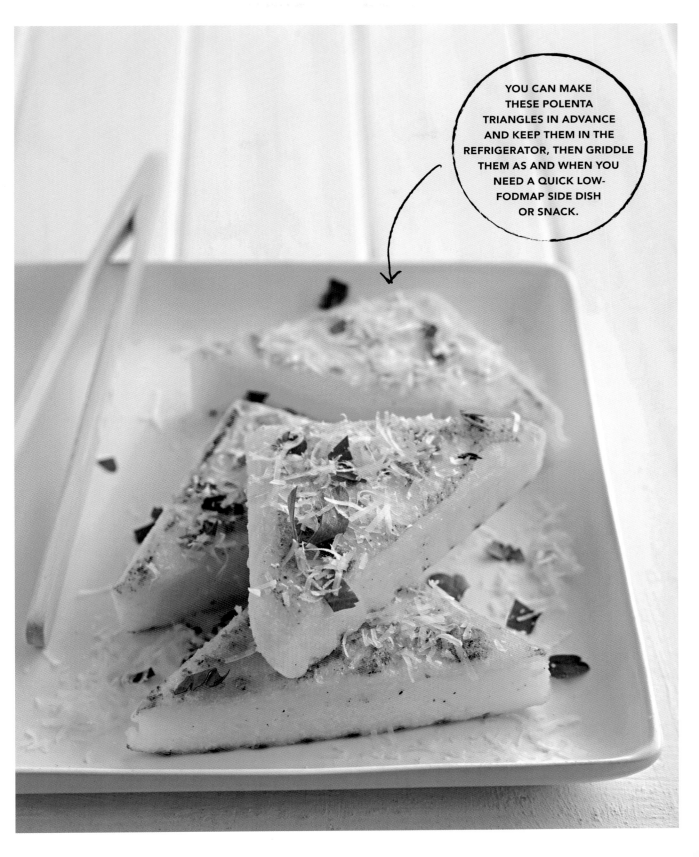

YOU CAN MAKE THESE POLENTA TRIANGLES IN ADVANCE AND KEEP THEM IN THE REFRIGERATOR, THEN GRIDDLE THEM AS AND WHEN YOU NEED A QUICK LOW-FODMAP SIDE DISH OR SNACK.

CARROT & PEPPER PILAF

**PREPARATION TIME: 20 MINUTES,
PLUS SOAKING AND STANDING
COOKING TIME: 20 MINUTES
SERVES: 4**

1¼ cups basmati rice

¼ cup sunflower oil

1 cinnamon stick

2 teaspoons cumin seeds

2 cloves

4 cardamom pods, lightly
bruised

8 black peppercorns

1 large carrot, peeled
and coarsely grated

2 cups sliced fresh or frozen
bell peppers

2 cups hot water

salt and freshly ground
black pepper

Wash the rice several times in cold water, then let it soak for
15 minutes. Drain thoroughly.

Heat the oil in a heavy saucepan. Add the spices and stir-fry for 2 to
3 minutes, until they release their aromas, then add the grated carrot
and pepper slices. Stir-fry for 2 to 3 minutes, until the vegetables are
well coated in the spicy oil, then add the rice. Stir the mixture as you
pour in the measured hot water. Season well.

Bring the mixture to a boil, cover the saucepan tightly with a lid,
reduce the heat, and simmer gently for 10 minutes. Do not lift the
lid to ensure you retain the steam inside the pan, which is required
for the cooking process.

Remove the pan from the heat and let stand, covered and
undisturbed, for 8 to 10 minutes. Fluff up the grains with a fork
and serve immediately.

1 tablespoon sunflower oil

2 eggplants, cut into cubes

1 red chile, seeded and thinly sliced, divided

2 teaspoons tamarind paste, divided

1 tablespoon dark brown sugar

2¾ cups cooked basmati rice

½ cup coarsely chopped mint leaves

7oz baby spinach

1 bunch of scallions (green parts only), thinly sliced

salt and freshly ground black pepper

TAMARIND CAN BE HIGH IN FODMAPS IF EATEN IN LARGER QUANTITIES, SO STICK TO THE QUANTITY STATED IN THIS RECIPE—USE NO MORE THAN ½ TEASPOON PER PORTION.

TAMARIND RICE

PREPARATION TIME: 10 MINUTES
COOKING TIME: ABOUT 15 MINUTES
SERVES: 4

Warm the oil in a large skillet over high heat. Add the cubed eggplant, half the sliced chile, 1 teaspoon of the tamarind paste, and the brown sugar. Stir-fry for 5 minutes, until the eggplant is golden and beginning to soften.

Add the cooked rice, mint, spinach, scallions, and the remaining tamarind to the eggplant. Stir-fry for a further 5 to 6 minutes or until piping hot.

Scatter with the remaining chile slices. Season with salt and pepper and serve immediately.

CAKES, BAKES & SWEET TREATS

SPICY CHARGRILLED PINEAPPLE →

Heat a ridged grill pan until very hot. Add the pineapple slices and cook until they start to caramelize, turning them over just once.

Add the maple syrup, chile flakes, and cinnamon and cook until the mixture starts to bubble. (This will not take long.)

Serve the pineapple slices drizzled with the spicy maple syrup and a dollop of yogurt.

PREPARATION TIME: 5 MINUTES
COOKING TIME: 10 MINUTES
SERVES: 4

8 slices of fresh pineapple, peeled and cored

1 tablespoon maple syrup

pinch of dried red chile flakes

pinch of ground cinnamon

plain lactose-free or plant-based yogurt (limit soy yogurt to ¼ cup per portion), or standard yogurt if you know you tolerate lactose

ORANGE BLOSSOM & ALMOND ORANGES

PREPARATION TIME: 10 MINUTES
SERVES: 4

4 large oranges

2 to 3 teaspoons orange blossom water

1 tablespoon confectioners' sugar

2 tablespoons almonds, coarsely chopped

Using a sharp knife, slice the tops and bases off the oranges, then remove the skin and pith. Slice each orange into 6 disks, reserving any juice.

Mix together the reserved juice, orange slices, orange blossom water (to taste), and confectioners' sugar in a bowl.

Divide the orange slices between 4 bowls, then drizzle the juice over each serving. Scatter with the almonds to serve.

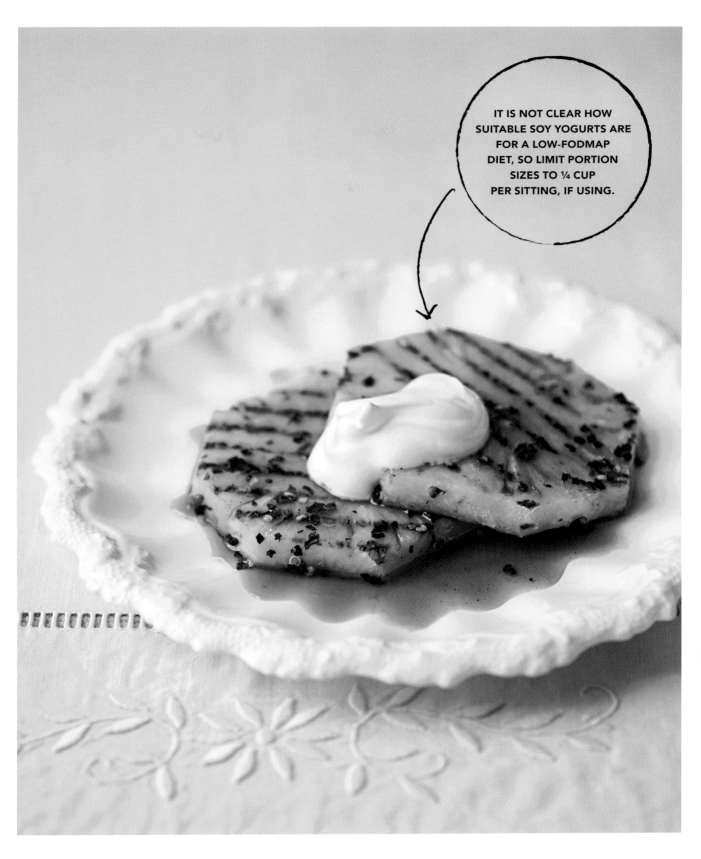

IT IS NOT CLEAR HOW SUITABLE SOY YOGURTS ARE FOR A LOW-FODMAP DIET, SO LIMIT PORTION SIZES TO ¼ CUP PER SITTING, IF USING.

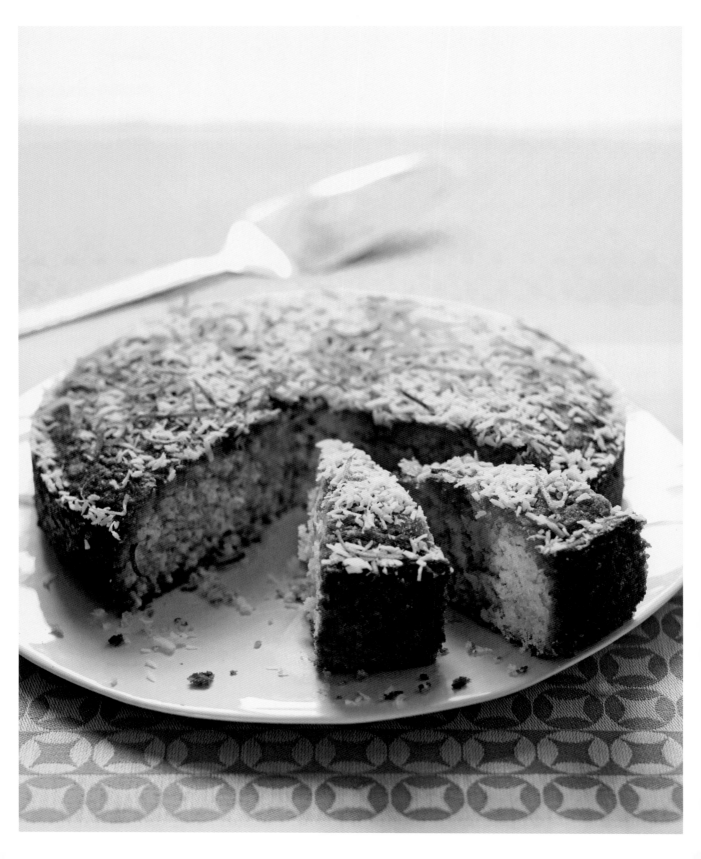

2 sticks unsalted butter, softened

1 cup superfine sugar

finely grated zest of 2 limes

3 eggs, lightly beaten

1²/₃ cups gluten-free self-rising flour, sifted

½ cup desiccated coconut

FOR THE TOPPING

¼ cup superfine sugar

juice of 2 limes

2 tablespoons desiccated coconut or freshly grated coconut

finely pared long strands of lime zest

LIME & COCONUT DRIZZLE CAKE

PREPARATION TIME: 20 MINUTES, PLUS COOLING
COOKING TIME: 35 TO 40 MINUTES
SERVES: 8

Preheat the oven to 350°F. Grease an 8-inch round springform cake pan and line the bottom with nonstick parchment paper.

Beat the butter, sugar, and grated lime zest together in a large bowl using a hand-held electric mixer until pale and fluffy. Beat in the eggs a little at a time, adding 1 tablespoon of the flour if the mixture starts to curdle, then fold in the flour and coconut with a large metal spoon.

Spoon the batter into the prepared pan and bake in the center of the oven for 35 to 40 minutes, until risen, golden, and shrinking away from the inside of the pan. Let cool in the pan.

While the cake is still warm, make the topping. Mix the sugar with the lime juice and drizzle the cake with the mixture. Scatter the cake with the coconut and strands of lime zest. Let cool completely before removing from the pan and slicing.

$1\frac{2}{3}$ cups gluten-free flour

2 eggs

$1\frac{1}{4}$ cups lactose-free or plant-based milk (limit soy to $\frac{1}{4}$ cup per portion), or standard milk if you know you tolerate lactose

$\frac{1}{2}$ tablespoon sunflower oil, for greasing

2 oranges

2 to 3 tablespoons superfine sugar, to serve

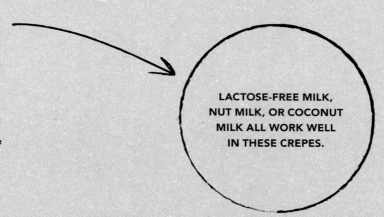

LACTOSE-FREE MILK, NUT MILK, OR COCONUT MILK ALL WORK WELL IN THESE CREPES.

SWEET ORANGE CREPES

PREPARATION TIME: 15 MINUTES, PLUS STANDING
COOKING TIME: 40 TO 60 MINUTES
SERVES: 4

Sift the flour into a bowl and make a well in the center. Add the eggs and beat, using a hand-held electric mixer, while gradually adding the milk, to incorporate the flour into the batter. Let stand for 10 minutes.

Heat a small, flat skillet over medium heat. Lightly oil it by wiping it with an oiled piece of paper towel. Pour a generous tablespoonful of the batter into the skillet and roll it around to completely coat the bottom. Cook for 3 to 4 minutes, then turn over and cook the other side for 2 to 3 minutes, until pale golden. Transfer the crepe to a sheet of parchment paper and keep warm. Repeat with the remaining batter to make 8 crepes.

Grate the orange zest, then segment the oranges, catching the juice. Pour the juice into another pan, add the segments and zest, and warm through. Divide the mixture into 8 portions and pour 1 of these over each crepe, then sprinkle with some superfine sugar to serve.

PREPARATION TIME: 10 MINUTES,
PLUS MARINATING
COOKING TIME: 5 TO 10 MINUTES
SERVES: 4

juice of 2 limes

⅓ cup superfine sugar

4 bananas, sliced into
3 to 4 pieces

1½ cups cornstarch

1 cup gluten-free
self-rising flour

3 tablespoons desiccated
coconut

3 large egg yolks

⅓ cup chilled soda water or
sparkling water

vegetable oil, for deep-frying

confectioners' sugar, for
dusting

maple syrup, for drizzling

LIME, BANANA & COCONUT FRITTERS

Preheat the oven to 300°F.

Mix together the lime juice and superfine sugar in a bowl. Add the bananas, stir well to coat, and let marinate for 5 minutes.

Roll the bananas in half the cornstarch until well coated and set aside.

Sift the remaining cornstarch and self-rising flour into a bowl. Stir in the coconut.

Whisk together the egg yolks and soda or sparkling water in a clean bowl. Add the flour mixture and whisk again until the mixture forms a thick batter.

Fill a deep medium-sized saucepan one-quarter full of vegetable oil. Heat the oil to 350°F or until a cube of bread immersed in the oil turns golden in 10 to 15 seconds.

Dip each piece of banana in the batter and carefully place it in the hot vegetable oil. Deep-fry in batches, for 1 to 2 minutes, until golden brown. Carefully remove the fritters from the oil using a slotted spoon and drain on paper towels. Keep the fritters warm on a plate in the warm oven while you fry the rest.

Serve immediately, dusted with confectioners' sugar and drizzled with maple syrup.

9oz strawberries, hulled and coarsely chopped

1 teaspoon finely grated lemon zest

1 to 2 teaspoons maple syrup, to taste

½ teaspoon vanilla bean paste or extract

2 teaspoons finely chopped mint (optional)

1 large egg white

¼ cup superfine sugar

> DON'T HAVE MORE THAN 1 SERVING OF THIS DISH AT A TIME TO REMAIN WITHIN THE FODMAP THRESHOLD—YOU SHOULD CONSUME NO MORE THAN 2¾OZ FRUIT PER SITTING.

INDIVIDUAL BAKED STRAWBERRY & LEMON MERINGUES

PREPARATION TIME: 20 MINUTES
COOKING TIME: 5 TO 7 MINUTES
SERVES: 4

Preheat the oven to 400°F.

Put the strawberries, lemon zest, maple syrup, vanilla bean paste, and chopped mint into a bowl and toss until all the ingredients are well combined. Spoon the strawberries and any liquid into 4 ramekins or other small, ovenproof dishes.

Place the egg white in a large, clean bowl and use a hand-held electric mixer to beat it until it forms firm peaks. Add the sugar, a tablespoon at a time, beating constantly, until all the sugar has been incorporated.

Spoon the raw meringue mixture in a high peak into each ramekin over the fruit, then bake for 5 to 7 minutes or until pale golden. Remove from the oven and serve immediately.

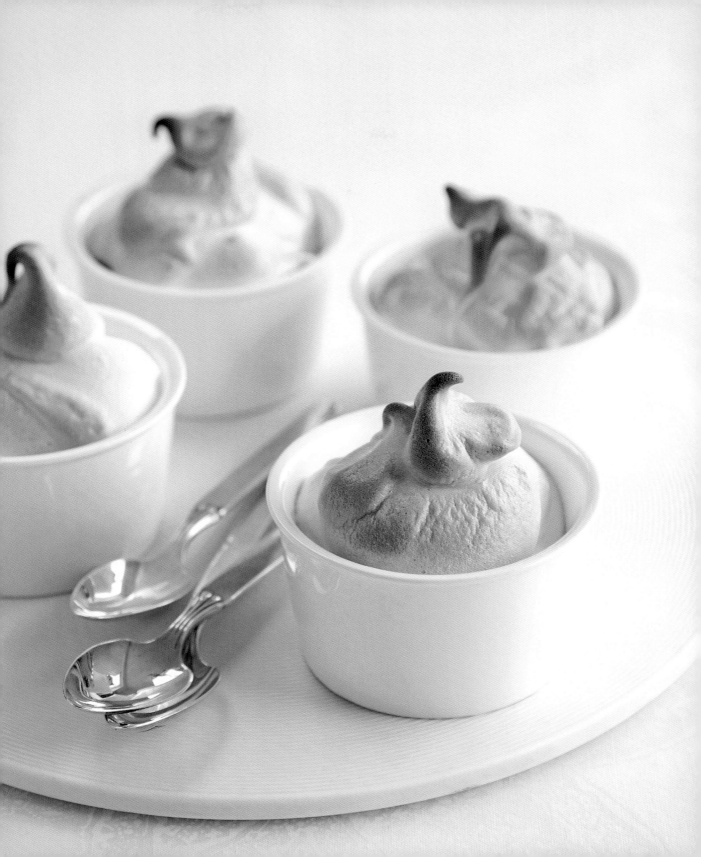

MELON, GINGER & LIME SORBET

**PREPARATION TIME: 15 MINUTES,
    PLUS CHURNING AND FREEZING
SERVES: 4**

1 large ripe Charentais melon
or Galia melon, chilled

¾ cup superfine sugar

1 tablespoon peeled and finely
grated fresh ginger root

juice of 2 limes

ice cream wafers, to serve

Cut the melon in half, remove and discard the seeds, then coarsely chop the flesh—you need about 1lb. Place it in a food processor with the sugar, ginger, and lime juice and blend until smooth.

Transfer the sorbet to an ice-cream maker and process following the manufacturer's instructions. Or, if you don't have an ice-cream maker, place the mixture in a freezerproof container and freeze for about 2 to 3 hours or until ice crystals have appeared on the surface. Beat with a hand-held electric beater until smooth, then return the mixture to the freezer. Repeat this process twice more until you have a fine-textured sorbet, then freeze until firm.

Remove the sorbet from the freezer 10 minutes before serving. Serve scooped into glasses, with a wafer.

- 1½ sticks butter, softened
- ¾ cup superfine sugar
- ½ cup rice flour
- ½ cup cornstarch
- 1 tablespoon baking powder
- grated zest and juice of 1 lemon
- 3 eggs, beaten
- 1 cup raspberries
- 1 tablespoon lemon curd (free from added fructose)

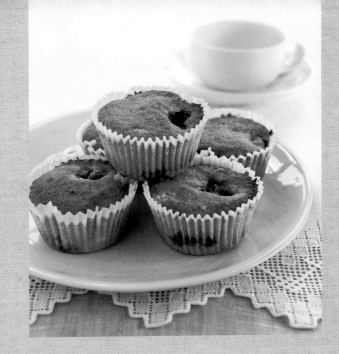

LEMON & RASPBERRY CUPCAKES

PREPARATION TIME: 15 MINUTES,
PLUS COOLING
COOKING TIME: 12 TO 15 MINUTES
MAKES: 12

Preheat the oven to 400°F. Line a large 12-hole muffin pan with paper muffin cups.

Beat together all the ingredients, except the raspberries and the lemon curd, in a large bowl. Fold in the raspberries.

Spoon half the batter into the prepared muffin cups. Dot each with a little of the lemon curd, then add the remaining batter on top.

Bake for 12 to 15 minutes, until golden and firm to the touch. Remove from the oven, transfer to a wire rack, and let cool.

2 cups gluten-free
self-rising flour
....
1 teaspoon gluten-free
baking powder
....
½ teaspoon baking soda
....
⅓ cup superfine sugar
....
½ cup desiccated coconut
....
½ stick unsalted
butter, melted
....
2 eggs
....
⅔ cup lactose-free or
plant-based milk (limit
soy to ¼ cup per portion),
or standard milk if you know
you tolerate lactose
....
1 cup raspberries

> YOU CAN USE FROZEN
> RASPBERRIES FOR THIS
> RECIPE IF FRESH BERRIES
> ARE OUT OF SEASON.

COCONUT & RASPBERRY MUFFINS

**PREPARATION TIME: 10 MINUTES,
PLUS COOLING**

COOKING TIME: 15 MINUTES

MAKES: 12

Preheat the oven to 400°F. Line a 12-hole muffin pan with paper muffin cups.

In a large bowl, sift together the flour, baking powder, and baking soda, then mix in the sugar and coconut. Make a well in the center of the mixture.

Beat together the melted butter, eggs, and milk in another bowl. Pour the wet ingredients into the dry ingredients and mix together gently, then fold in the raspberries when the batter is nearly combined—do not overmix.

Spoon the batter into the paper muffin cups. Bake for 15 minutes, until golden and slightly risen. Transfer to a wire rack to cool.

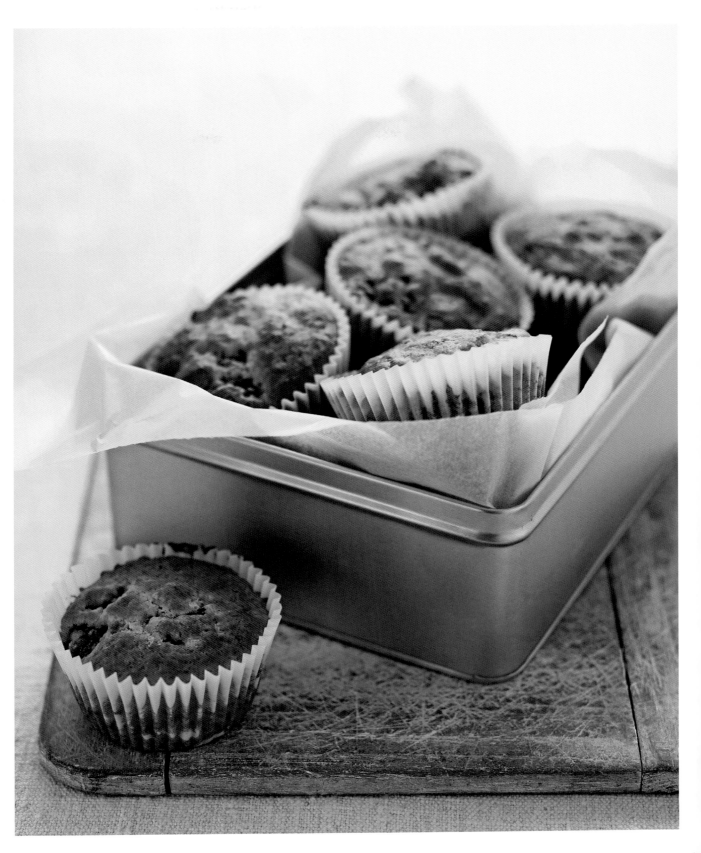

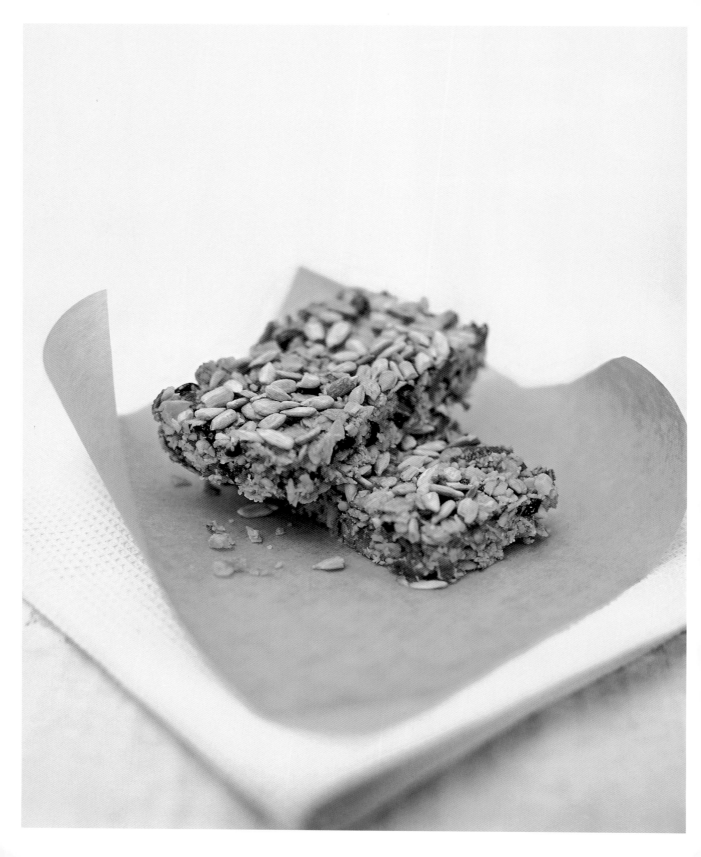

1 stick butter, plus extra for greasing

¼ cup maple syrup

2 tablespoons soft light brown sugar

2 cups rolled oats

¾ cup oatmeal

¾ cup chopped mixed low-FODMAP nuts (such as walnuts, peanuts, and macadamia nuts)

⅓ cup dried blueberries

2 tablespoons sunflower seeds

IF YOU ARE FOLLOWING A GLUTEN-FREE DIET FOR CELIAC OR GLUTEN SENSITIVITY, YOU WILL NEED TO CHOOSE GLUTEN-FREE OATS.

FRUIT & NUT BARS

PREPARATION TIME: 10 MINUTES, PLUS COOLING
COOKING TIME: 18 TO 20 MINUTES
MAKES: 8

Preheat the oven to 400°F. Grease an 8-inch square nonstick baking pan lightly and line the bottom with nonstick parchment paper.

Melt the butter, syrup, and sugar together in a saucepan. Stir in the remaining ingredients, except the sunflower seeds, then press the mixture into the prepared pan.

Sprinkle with the sunflower seeds, then bake for 15 minutes or until golden. Cut into 8 bars and let cool.

PREPARATION TIME: 20 MINUTES
COOKING TIME: 35 TO 45 MINUTES
SERVES: 8 TO 10

butter, for greasing

4 egg whites

¼ teaspoon cream of tartar

½ cup firmly packed light brown sugar

½ cup superfine sugar

1 teaspoon white wine vinegar

½ cup walnut pieces, lightly toasted and chopped

FOR THE FILLING

1 cup heavy whipping cream

9oz strawberries

STRAWBERRY MACAROON CAKE

Preheat the oven to 300°F. Grease 2 x 8-inch cake pans and then line the bottoms with nonstick parchment paper.

Beat the egg whites and cream of tartar in a large clean bowl until stiff. Combine the sugars in a bowl, then gradually beat the sugars into the egg white a little at a time, until fully incorporated. Add the vinegar and beat for a few minutes more until the meringue mixture is thick and glossy. Fold in the walnuts.

Divide the meringue mixture evenly between the prepared cake pans. Level off the surfaces, then swirl the tops with the back of a spoon. Bake for 35 to 45 minutes, until lightly browned and crisp. Use a sharp knife to loosen the edges of the meringues in the pans, then let cool in the pans.

Re-loosen the edges of the meringues, then turn out each meringue onto a clean dish cloth. Peel off the lining papers. Set 1 of the meringues onto a serving plate.

Whip the cream to soft peaks, then spoon three-quarters of the whipped cream over the meringue on the serving plate. Halve 8 of the smallest strawberries and set aside. Hull and slice the remaining berrries and arrange them on the layer of cream. Cover with the second meringue, ensuring the top of this meringue layer is facing upward. Decorate with spoonfuls of the remaining cream and the reserved halved strawberries. Serve within 2 hours of assembly.

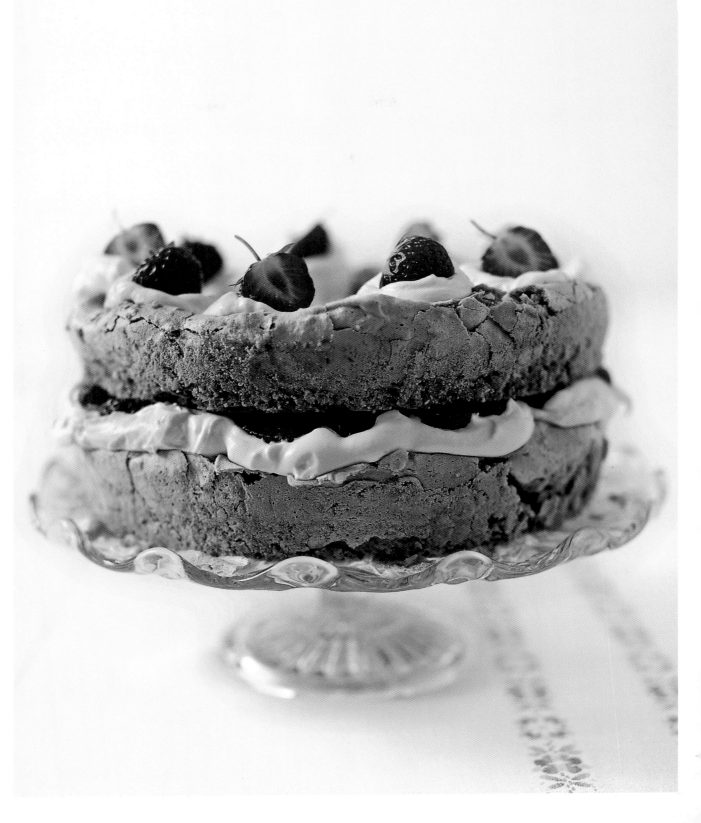

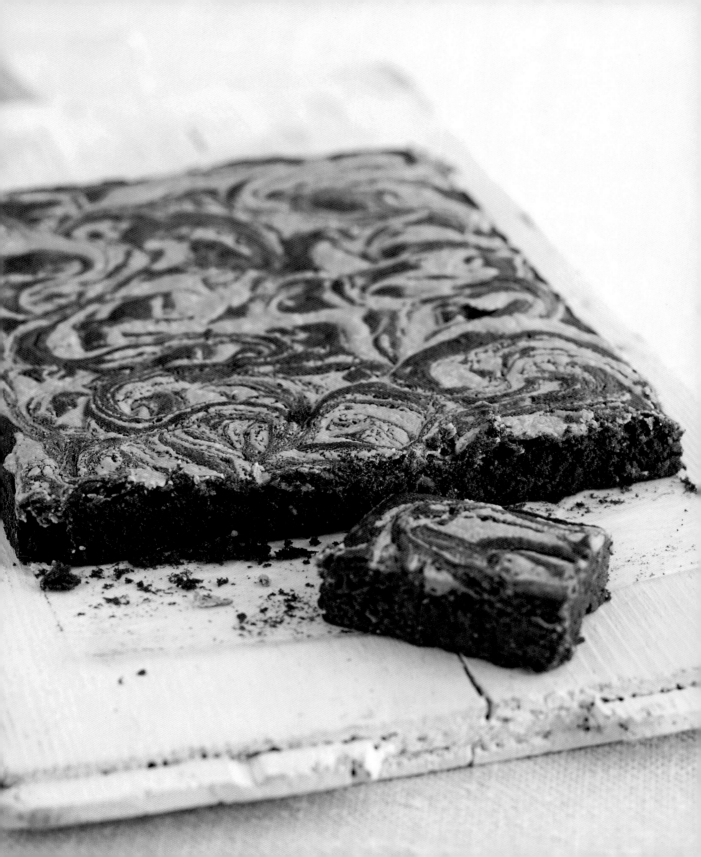

1½ sticks unsalted butter, plus extra for greasing

7oz dark chocolate, broken into small pieces

⅓ cup crunchy peanut butter (free from high-fructose corn syrup)

½ cup smooth peanut butter (free from high-fructose corn syrup)

3 large eggs

1 cup superfine sugar

¼ teaspoon salt

½ cup gluten-free self-rising flour

PEANUT BUTTER SWIRL BROWNIES

PREPARATION TIME: 10 MINUTES
COOKING TIME: 30 MINUTES
MAKES: 12 TO 16

Preheat the oven to 400°F. Grease a 12 x 8 inch baking pan and line it with nonstick parchment paper.

Put the butter, chocolate, and crunchy peanut butter into a small saucepan over low heat and warm until just melted. In a separate saucepan, gently warm through the smooth peanut butter.

Meanwhile, put the eggs, sugar, and salt into a large bowl and beat until combined. Using a rubber spatula, stir in the melted chocolate mixture and flour.

Scrape the mixture into the prepared pan. Drizzle with the smooth peanut butter in 3 to 4 straight lines, then drag the tip of a sharp knife through the peanut butter to create a marbled effect.

Bake for 18 to 20 minutes, until the cake is just firm to the touch, but has a slightly fudgy texture. Let cool in the pan for 1 to 2 minutes, then lift out the block onto a cutting board using the lining paper and cut it into 12 to 16 squares. Serve warm or cold.

1 stick unsalted
butter, softened

¼ cup superfine sugar

grated zest of 1 orange

¼ cup unsweetened cocoa
powder

½ cup gluten-free
all-purpose flour

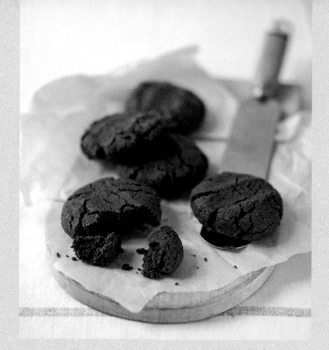

CHOCOLATE ORANGE SHORTBREAD

**PREPARATION TIME: 10 MINUTES,
PLUS CHILLING AND COOLING
COOKING TIME: 15 MINUTES
SERVES: 4**

Preheat the oven to 375°F. Line a cookie sheet with nonstick parchment paper.

Cream together the butter, sugar, and orange zest in a large bowl until the mixture is light and fluffy.

Mix in the cocoa powder and flour and bring the mixture together into a ball of dough. Cover the bowl with plastic wrap and let chill for 10 minutes.

Shape the mixture into walnut-sized balls and place these on the prepared cookie sheet, ensuring they are well spaced. Bake for 5 minutes. Remove the cookie sheet from the oven and lightly press down each ball of dough with your finger. Return the shortbread to the oven and bake for a further 5 to 7 minutes, until it has started to become crisp on top.

Transfer to a wire rack and let cool completely.

5½oz dark chocolate
(85 percent cocoa solids),
broken into pieces

½ cup coconut cream

1 tablespoon mint leaves

1 cup raspberries

½ teaspoon unsweetened
cocoa powder

½ teaspoon confectioners'
sugar

COCONUT CREAM, LIKE
COCONUT MILK, SHOULD BE
LIMITED TO ½ CUP ON THE
LOW-FODMAP DIET.

ULTRA-RICH CHOCOLATE STACKS

**PREPARATION TIME: 20 MINUTES,
   PLUS CHILLING
SERVES: 4**

Line a cookie sheet with nonstick parchment paper.

Put the chocolate pieces into a heatproof bowl and set it over a saucepan of gently simmering water, ensuring the water does not touch the base of the bowl. Stir the chocolate until melted.

Spoon 12 spoonfuls of the melted chocolate onto the prepared cookie sheet and allow each to spread into a disk measuring about 2¾ inches in diameter. Refrigerate for 30 minutes until set.

Whip the coconut cream in a bowl until thick. Layer 3 chocolate disks on each of 4 serving plates with the coconut cream, mint leaves, and raspberries.

Mix the cocoa and confectioner's sugar together, then dust the mixture over the chocolate stacks to serve.

1¹/₂ sticks butter, softened, plus extra for greasing

1 cup superfine sugar

1 cup brown rice flour, plus extra for dusting

3 eggs

1 tablespoon baking powder

few drops of vanilla extract

1 tablespoon lactose-free or plant-based milk (limit soy to ¹/₄ cup per portion), or standard milk if you know you tolerate lactose

TO DECORATE

¹/₄ cup raspberry jam

confectioner's sugar

VICTORIA SPONGE CAKE

PREPARATION TIME: 10 MINUTES, PLUS COOLING
COOKING TIME: 20 MINUTES
SERVES: 12

Preheat the oven to 400°F. Grease and flour 2 x 7-inch round cake pans.

Put all the cake ingredients into the bowl of a food processor and whizz until smooth. (Or, beat the ingredients together in a large bowl until the mixture is light and fluffy.)

Spoon the mixture into the prepared pans and bake for about 20 minutes, until risen and golden. Transfer to a wire rack to cool.

Sandwich the cooled cakes together with the jam and dust with confectioners' sugar.

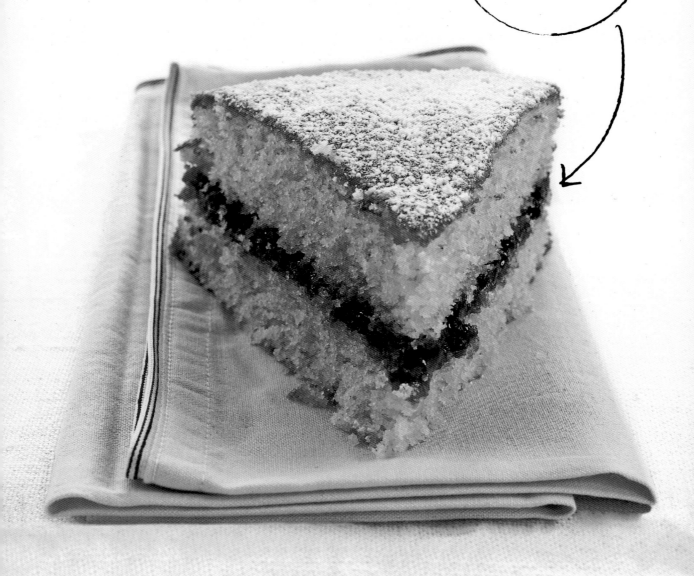

10½oz good-quality dark chocolate with chile (70 percent cocoa solids), broken into pieces

1½ sticks unsalted butter, diced

6 eggs, separated

½ cup superfine sugar

FOR THE CHILE SYRUP

1 red chile, seeded and thinly sliced

grated zest and juice of 1 lime

½ cup superfine sugar

⅔ cup water

HIGH-FAT FOODS CAN CAUSE A FLARE-UP IN GASTROINTESTINAL SYMPTOMS, EVEN IF THEY ARE LOW IN FODMAPS, SO STICK TO A MODERATE SLIVER OF THIS DELICIOUS DESSERT.

CHOCOLATE & CHILE MOUSSE CAKE

PREPARATION TIME: 20 MINUTES, PLUS COOLING AND CHILLING
COOKING TIME: 35 MINUTES
SERVES: 8 TO 10

Preheat the oven to 350°F. Line the bottom of an 8-inch springform cake pan with nonstick parchment paper.

Melt the chocolate and butter in a heatproof bowl set over a saucepan of gently simmering water, stirring the chocolate occasionally, ensuring the water does not touch the base of the bowl.

Meanwhile, whisk the egg yolks with the sugar in a bowl until pale and thick. Stir in the melted chocolate mixture.

Beat the egg whites in a separate large, grease-free bowl until they form soft peaks. Using a metal spoon, fold a couple of tablespoons of the egg white into the chocolate mixture to loosen it, then fold in the remaining egg white. Pour the mixture into the prepared pan and bake for 20 minutes. Remove the pan from the oven, cover it with kitchen foil (to prevent a crust from forming), and let cool. Chill in the refrigerator for at least 4 hours or overnight.

To make the syrup, combine all the ingredients in a small saucepan and heat over low heat, stirring, until the sugar has dissolved. Bring to a boil, then simmer for 10 minutes, until syrupy. Let cool.

Remove the cake from the refrigerator 30 minutes before serving in slices, drizzled with the syrup.

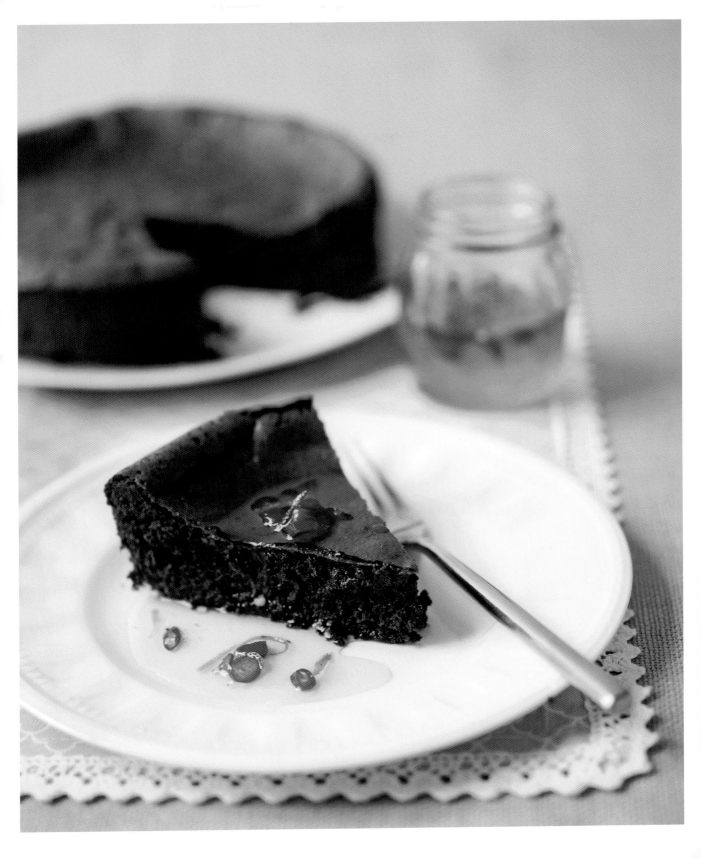

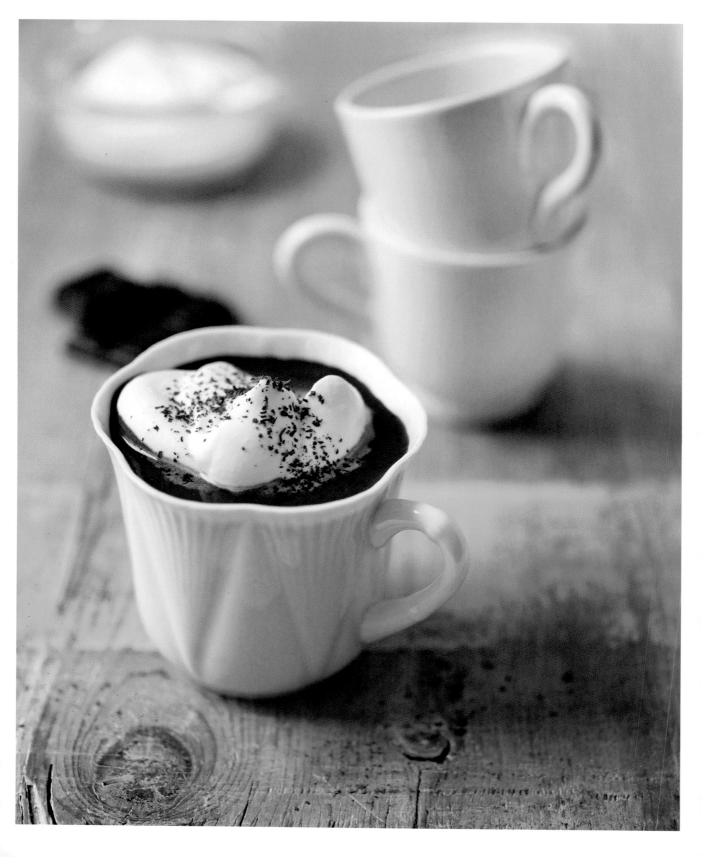

IF USING COCONUT MILK, REDUCE THE QUANTITY TO ½ CUP PER PORTION. LACTOSE-FREE MILKS CAN BE ENJOYED IN UNLIMITED AMOUNTS.

6oz dark chocolate, broken into pieces

1 large pinch of chili powder

2 tablespoons superfine sugar

2 large pinches of ground cinnamon

2 vanilla beans, split lengthwise

2½ cups milk, or lactose-free or plant-based milk (due to recommended portion limitations you cannot substitute soy milk for this recipe)

1 cup heavy whipping cream, whipped

grated dark chocolate, to serve (limit each portion to 1½oz)

CHILE HOT CHOCOLATE

PREPARATION TIME: 10 MINUTES
COOKING TIME: 5 MINUTES
SERVES: 4

Place the chocolate, chili powder, sugar, cinnamon, vanilla beans, and milk into a pan and heat gently until the chocolate has melted. Bring the mixture to a boil and whisk until the chocolate is very smooth and frothy. Remove the vanilla beans.

Pour the chocolate into 4 warmed mugs and top with the whipped cream and grated chocolate.

INDEX

RESOURCES

USEFUL INFORMATION

King's College London, UK
Information on the low-FODMAP diet from one of the world's leading research and teaching universities:
www.kcl.ac.uk/lsm/research/divisions/dns/projects/fodmaps/faq.aspx

Monash University, Australia
Information on the low-FODMAP diet from the medical researchers who first developed it:
www.med.monash.edu/cecs/gastro/fodmap/

The Irritable Bowel Syndrome Self Help and Support Group
A US-based "trusted community for IBS and digestive health sufferers":
www.ibsgroup.org

FIND A DIETITIAN

When looking for a dietitian, check with the individual practitioner that they are able to advise on the low-FODMAP diet.

For a dietitian specializing in the low-FODMAP diet worldwide:
fodmap-diet.com/find-a-fodmap-dietitian/

For a registered dietitian in America:
www.eatright.org/find-an-expert

For a registered dietitian in Canada:
www.dietitians.ca/Your-Health/Find-A-Dietitian/Find-a-Dietitian.aspx

For a registered dietitian in Australia:
daa.asn.au/find-an-apd/

For a registered dietitian in New Zealand:
dietitians.org.nz/find-a-dietitian/

For a registered dietitian in Ireland:
https://www.indi.ie/find-a-dietitian.html

THE REINTRODUCTION PHASE

Re-challenging and Reintroducing FODMAPs: A self-help guide to the entire reintroduction phase of the low FODMAP diet by Lee Martin (CreateSpace Independent Publishing Platform, 2016).
A useful guide to the reintroduction phase of the low-FODMAP diet.

APPS

The Monash University Low FODMAP Diet
Developed for use by researchers at Monash University, Australia, this app assists in the management of the gastrointestinal symptoms associated with IBS. It works on a traffic light system to indicate which foods are suitable for a low-FODMAP diet.

ACKNOWLEDGMENTS

I would like to thank the team at King's College London for heading up such fantastic work on the research and dissemination of the low-FODMAP diet in the UK. I know you all work so hard to design and undertake clinical trials, train dietitians and develop resources to help health professionals and patients get the most out of the low-FODMAP diet. It was the team at King's College London who put FODMAPs on my radar back in the late 2000s and I have since learned so much from their expertise and their published research.

I would also like to thank Imperial College NHS Trust for supporting me from the very beginning in setting up a low-FODMAP service and run a dedicated clinic to help those with functional bowel disorders.

Thank you to Octopus Publishing who have worked so hard on this book and got it to print in such a short time frame.

Last but definitely not least I would like to thank my patients whom I admire so much for working so hard to improve their symptoms: seeing you improve brings me so much joy – I am constantly learning from you.

PICTURE CREDITS